Springer Series on Medical Education

Steven Jonas, MD, Foun<
Carol J. Bland, PhD, Se1

D1388721

Jane Westberg, PhD, has devoted almost 30 years to finding ways to enhance and humanize the processes of teaching and learning in the health professions. Currently she is Clinical Professor in the Department of Family Medicine at the University of Colorado School of Medicine and Associate Editor of *Education for Health*. She has served on the faculties of the University of Miami School of Medicine and George Washington University School of Medicine. She and her colleague and husband, Hill Jason, have been consultants to scores of institutions nationally and internationally and have conducted hundreds of workshops and seminars for health professions educators. Jane is senior author of five previous books coauthored by Hill: *Making Presentations* (1991); *Providing Constructive Feedback* (1992); *Collaborative Clinical Education: The Foundation of Effective Health Care* (1993); *Teaching Creatively with Video* (1994); and *Fostering Learning in Small Groups* (1996). Jane has written numerous articles, chapters, and instructional materials for health professionals and has written and produced more than 40 nationally distributed educational video programs. She has also written extensively about Native Americans in the health professions for *Winds of Change* magazine. Jane and Hill have four children and two grandchildren.

Since the late 1950s **Hilliard Jason, MD, EdD,** has devoted his career to finding ways to help enhance the quality of teaching in the health professions. He was founding Director of the Office of Medical Education Research and Development (OMERAD) at Michigan State University's College of Human Medicine (1966–72), the Division of Faculty Development at the Association of American Medical Colleges (1974–78), and the National Center for Faculty Development at the University of Miami School of Medicine (1978–90). He is now Clinical Professor of Family Medicine at the University of Colorado School of Medicine and editor of *Education for Health: Change in Learning and Practice,* the journal of The Network: Community Partnerships for Health through Innovative Education, Service, and Research. He is senior author of *Teachers and Teaching in U.S. Medical Schools* (1982), a book coauthored by his wife, Jane Westberg. He has also written many articles, chapters, and instructional materials in the areas of faculty development and medical teaching. Hill has been the executive producer, cowriter, and host of more than 50 educational video programs in the health professions and an educational consultant in 29 countries.

Contents

Introduction

Helping learners in the health professions become thoughtful, competent practitioners is an enormous challenge. Helping them develop the attitudes and skills needed to continually enhance and update their knowledge and skills in the rapidly changing world of health care is especially daunting.

After decades of working with educators, students, residents, and practitioners in the health professions, we've become convinced that there are two key ways to help others learn from experience and thereby get the most out of their formal education and continue to learn effectively throughout their careers. First, we must help them become reflective practitioners who regularly think about and assess their work and invite the reflections and feedback of others. Second, we must give them timely, constructive feedback on their work and self-assessments.

This book is for our colleagues—physicians, nurses, psychologists, social workers, basic scientists, and others—who are full-time or part-time educators of students, residents, and practitioners in the health professions. The underlying principles and many of the strategies that we discuss could also be of interest to educators in other fields.

We define *reflection* and briefly describe the reflective practitioner. Then we examine the rationale for fostering reflection and providing feedback and explore some barriers to accomplishing these tasks. Later we offer practical steps to consider taking when helping learners become reflective practitioners. We also suggest strategies for directly providing feedback to learners and for helping them get constructive feedback from patients and other learners.

Reflection and feedback need to be based on experiences. Learning begins when people engage in activities in which they make choices and perform tasks. Typically they *do* something: gather and critically review information, solve a problem, communicate with patients. The kinds of experiences we use as examples range from classroom settings where students role-play and work through paper-based cases to clinical and community settings where students care for and learn from patients and their families. The situations we describe include educators working with groups of learners and educators doing one-on-one precepting. If our examples don't fit the kind of teaching you do, please adapt what we've written to the work that you do. If you don't currently engage your students in tasks that relate to their future clinical work , we hope we can convince you to do so.

We realize that teachers who are working in environments that devalue reflection may find it difficult to help learners become reflective practitioners. In the epilogue we provide a few suggestions for teachers in this situation.

This book grew out of a book that is now out of print titled *Providing Constructive Feedback* (Westberg & Jason, 1991). The current book also derives from our experiences offering courses, workshops, and seminars, most of which have included some focus on reflection and feedback. In addition, some of the material is an extension of parts of our books dealing with clinical supervision (Westberg & Jason, 1993), teaching with video (Westberg & Jason, 1994b), and fostering learning in small groups (Westberg & Jason, 1996).

We gratefully acknowledge our many colleagues from whom we have learned so much. We particularly thank those who reviewed this manuscript and provided us with valuable, constructive feedback. They are Steven Jonas, MD, founding editor of the Springer Series on Medical Education; Rick Botelho, MD; Ronald Epstein, MD; Michael Gordon, PhD; and Savina Schoenhofer, PhD, RN.

CHAPTER 1

Why Foster Reflection?

It is often said that patients are the best teachers for health professionals. We agree that experiences in caring for patients and families can provide rich learning opportunities, as can clinically relevant exercises and experiences in classrooms. In fact, direct experiences in which learners practice the skills they need as practitioners are the foundation for meaningful learning. Schools in the health professions should provide more of these experiences and offer them earlier than most now do. Engaging in significant tasks is a key to learning, but the old aphorism "practice makes perfect" is incomplete. Experience alone does not automatically result in desirable, lasting learning.

Our work with learners and the contributions of many colleagues have convinced us that in order for students, residents, and practitioners to learn from their experiences (during their formal education and for the rest of their careers), they need to be reflective *during* and *after* these experiences. Particularly when working on new skills, when trying to make substantial changes in established skills, and when dealing with difficult patient-care challenges, learners can benefit from the reflections and feedback of others. In this chapter we discuss what it means to be reflective as a learner and practitioner and why reflection is one of the keys to learning from experience and providing high-quality health care. In the next chapter we explore feedback, another critical key to learning.

To be reflective is to have a heightened awareness during and after experiences and to be eager to learn from them. As regularly as they can during important experiences, reflective learners and practitioners try to be attentive to their feelings and thoughts, to the choices that are available to them, to what they know or don't know that is relevant to the situation, and to the apparent effectiveness or ineffectiveness of what they are doing. When the experience involves patients, reflective students and practitioners also try to be aware of the uniqueness of that person and the interpersonal dynamics of the encounter.

Schön (1983, 1987) reminds us that we can reflect *in* action, and we can reflect *on* action. When learners and practitioners are reflecting in action while caring for a patient, they function on two levels: They are engaged in the tasks at hand, such as eliciting information or giving bad news, and they are observing, questioning, and assessing the tasks in which they are engaged, making continuous adjustments in what they do according to what they discern about the process. Once the task is concluded, they remain reflective—that is, reflect *on* action—particularly if there were surprises, troubling events, or unanswered questions. As we'll discuss, reflecting in and on their actions enables students and practitioners to be continually learning from experience, ultimately enabling them to provide high-quality patient care.

Why should schools and residency programs provide time in their curricula for reflection, including self-assessment? Why is it desirable for learners to develop the habit of reflecting on their experiences? Why should teachers be asked to work with learners on these skills? Why should we strive to help our learners become reflective practitioners? These are the question we seek to answer in the remainder of this chapter.

REASONS FOR FOSTERING REFLECTION

Too many health-profession learners do not have well-developed reflection skills.   Many learners in the health professions live in cultures in which "doing" and "being productive" are highly valued, and quiet reflection is neglected or devalued. Radios, televisions, amplified music, people talking on cell phones, and other sources of noise are so pervasive that even people who want to be reflective can find it difficult to do so. Not surprisingly, most students have had little practice reflecting on their experiences.

Self-assessment is an important component of reflection. Research in health-profession education indicates that students do not know intuitively how to engage in systematic self-assessment (Gordon, 1997). Most students' self-assessment skills are weak and are not developed and improved by conventional clinical education (Gordon, 1991). Some learners fail to recognize their shortcomings. Others are more critical of their performance than are their teachers (Stuart, Goldstein, & Snope, 1980; Wondrak & Goble, 1992). When students do not learn the skills of self-assessment, their assessments of their knowledge and performance can be potentially misleading extensions of their global self-concepts (Gordon, 1992).

The skills of reflection, including self-assessment, can be learned. To become reflective learners and practitioners, students and residents need teachers who help them understand the meaning and importance of reflection. As with learning any complex skill, students and residents must want to develop the habits of mind and the skills required for being reflective. They also need many opportunities to practice reflecting on experiences, to reflect on the experience of being reflective, and to receive feedback on their efforts from teachers and others.

All of this depends on learners having role models they respect who regularly are reflective. They also need sufficient time for reflection and worthy experiences on which to reflect. These experiences, which can be either real or simulated, need to involve learners in clinically relevant tasks such as assessing patients' needs, problem-solving (alone or with colleagues), gathering and critically reviewing pertinent literature, wrestling with ethical issues, developing treatment plans, and communicating effectively with patients. Simulated experiences that give learners practice in using clinical skills include role-playing and problem-based learning (PBL). (In PBL small groups of learners engage in problem-solving and other clinical activities as they work through a case, usually a patient-care situation. For detailed descriptions of PBL, see Barrows & Tamblyn, 1980; Barrows, 1985; and Westberg & Jason, 1996.)

Gordon's research (1991, 1992, 1999) documents that the self-assessment component of reflection can be learned. The accuracy and validity of students' self-assessments improve when the students understand and practice the skills involved in systematically gathering and interpreting data on their work and receive feedback on their progress by comparing and reconciling their independent assessments of their performance with assessments done by teachers.

Reflection enables learners to identify and build on their existing knowledge.   People learn by identifying and building new knowledge on their existing knowledge (Whitman, 1993). When learners reflect on experiences they have in the classroom, in the community, and in patient-care settings, they can clarify what they already know so that their existing knowledge, including life experiences, can better serve as a foundation on which to build new knowledge. For example, in problem-based learning, students who are trying to understand the etiology of a patient's condition reflect on what they already know that they can bring to bear on the case. Then they share what they know with the other members of their group. This process gives learners a foundation on which to construct the new understanding that derives from working on this case and helps them gain some self-confidence from realizing that they already know something about health care.

Reflection can enable learners to identify deficits in their knowledge and errors in their thinking.   As learners reflect on experiences, such as trying to solve paper-based clinical challenges or real patient-care problems, they can discover what they already know. And they can bump up against what they don't know and need to learn. They can make many of these discoveries on their own. With the help of teachers or others who facilitate their reflection, they can make additional discoveries. Once learners identify what they need to work on, they can develop and feel ownership of a set of meaningful learning goals and plans for achieving those goals.

Reflection can enable learners to generalize from particular experiences and apply this new knowledge in later situations. Kolb (1984) proposes that the ideal learning cycle proceeds from concrete experiences to observations and reflections, then to the formulation of abstract concepts and generalizations, and finally to testing the implications of these concepts in new situations. For example, as a student reflects with her preceptor on a videotape of an encounter she just had with a patient, she realizes that the yes-or-no questions she was asking the patient made it difficult for him to tell his story. However, when she used an open-ended question, the patient's more complete response included several important details about his problem that she might otherwise have missed. After a discussion with her preceptor, the student makes the generalization that open-ended questions can enable patients to tell their stories in a fuller, richer way. The next time she does a history on a patient, she plans to begin with open-ended questions, following up with more focused questions for eliciting missing details. Without reflection, students are less likely to form generalizations or achieve carry over to new settings.

Reflection can help learners integrate new understanding. Experiences can lead to insights that can be lost if learners rush to their next experience without taking time to explore their new insight further. Taking time for reflection, alone or with others, enables learners to elaborate on fresh insights, connect them with what they know, link them with other knowledge areas, derive generalizations, and figure out how they can use these insights in other situations, as we described above. All of this helps create a web—a structure—of deep, rich connections that help learners make these new understandings truly their own.

With reflection, including self-assessment, learning can be accelerated. Sports coaches have long known that athletes' rates of improvement accelerate if they spend some of their time reviewing and critiquing their performance and "metabolizing" what happened instead of using all of their time practicing. Following some practice sessions and most competitions, elite athletes routinely review and critique their performances, often using videotaped recordings of their performance as an aid. This reflection on ("processing" of) performance has met with similar success in the education of physicians (Jason, Kagan, Werner, Elstein, & Thomas, 1971; Kahn, Cohen, & Jason, 1979), physician's assistants (Westberg, Kahn, Cohen, & Friel, 1980), nurses (DeTornyay & Thompson, 1982), and mental health professionals (Kagan & Kagan, 1991).

Reflection can enable learners to identify unexamined assumptions and biases that can interfere with learning and patient care. All of us have assumptions and biases, which can lead to distorted impressions and faulty conclusions. A student who thinks that most addicts are street people might miss the fact that his well-groomed, wealthy patient has an addiction. The learner might discover the inaccuracy of his assumption through his own reflection, or he might need the help of a teacher who can assist him in questioning the validity of his assumption. Ideally, the teacher will also help him be aware that he, like other learners and practitioners, may be operating on the basis of incorrect assumptions in other patient-care situations. By helping him become routinely vigilant about the risk of bias and unfounded assumptions, the teacher can introduce the learner to a pattern of being appropriately reflective and of being open to others who may help him see aspects of his own behavior that will interfere with learning and patient care.

Reflection can enable learners to be in touch with their feelings so they can take care of themselves and provide compassionate, comprehensive care. The process of becoming a health care practitioner is stressful. Studying for exams, dissecting a cadaver, witnessing children who have been abused, caring for patients of their own age who are seriously ill or disabled, or making a mistake when caring for patients can evoke strong feelings in learners. If students have opportunities to acknowledge and reflect on these feelings, the result can be personal growth. However, when learners don't have opportunities to recognize and process strong feelings and disturbing events, there is a risk that they will bury their feelings or express them in undesirable ways, including putting up inappropriate barriers between themselves and patients and avoiding emotionally charged situations. For example, a student who is not helped to work through his painful feelings about his first patient death might develop a pattern (as too many health professionals now do) of avoiding contact with patients who are dying. He may even not talk with dying patients about crucial issues that need attention, such as medical options that are available to them during their remaining months of life.

If learners are to become empathic, compassionate practitioners, they need to get to know themselves and to be reasonably comfortable with who they are. Otherwise, they may not be able to empathize with patients or even provide adequate care. A student who blames herself for having been sexually abused as a child and is unable to think about those early events is not likely to be able to be fully empathic and compassionate with a patient who was sexually abused. She also may not refer the abused patient for counseling or other needed care and may avoid asking other patients questions about possible abuse experiences or sexual issues in their lives.

Learners who tune into their feelings, while with patients and afterwards, can learn a great deal about themselves. This can include becoming aware of those situations that they can't handle alone because of their own unresolved issues.

Learners are likely to feel more ownership of insights that emerge from their own discoveries. After observing learners examining a patient or engaging in another activity, teachers may be tempted to offer their insights and feedback, especially if they feel that as a teacher they are expected to do so. However, when teachers present their insights and feedback without allowing learners to do their own thinking, they risk robbing the learners of opportunities to make their own discoveries. In fact, if teachers repeatedly interject their reflections and feedback prematurely, some learners may stop being reflective, lose confidence in their own perceptions, and become increasingly dependent on teachers for ideas and answers. Others who are cut off by teachers may feel demeaned, become angry, and stop listening to their teachers. Neither group of learners is likely to feel ownership of what their teachers tell them. Learners who make their own discoveries about their work—even disappointing discoveries—are more likely to acknowledge and own these discoveries than if these insights are pointed out by others (Dewey, 1938).

Learners can feel more self-respect and confidence if they identify their deficiencies and strengths. Like most people, learners feel uncomfortable when they receive negative feedback. When we withhold our feedback until learners have assessed their performance, they can be the first to identify their problem areas, enabling them to have a greater sense of dignity and self-respect, which can help them develop confidence in their perceptions and judgments. If we succeed in establishing trust-based relationships with learners, they will be less likely to "edit" what they reveal to us and may point out some of the very problems we had intended to identify. Learners may even reveal problems we hadn't noticed. We are then in the pleasant position of being able to give them positive feedback on their perceptive self-assessment (Westberg & Jason, 1994a).

Learners' reflections can focus us more accurately on what they need. When learners reflect aloud on their work, they often provide invaluable "diagnostic" information about both the *content* of their reflection (for instance, issues they regard as important and the extent to which they understand these issues) and their command of the *process* of reflection (such as their capacities as communicators, their comfort with reflecting on their work, and the accuracy and subtleties of their self-assessments). This information enables us to tailor what we say and do to our learners' unique strengths and needs.

Inviting learners' reflections can help us foster collaborative relationships with them. As we argue extensively elsewhere, students are likely to learn more quickly and effectively if they are active partners in their education rather than the mere recipients of our presentations (Westberg & Jason, 1993, 1994b, 1996). Traditionally, the relationship between teachers and learners has been based on an authoritarian model in which teachers do things for and to learners. Not surprisingly, the relationships between our graduates (especially physicians) and their patients have also tended toward being authoritarian. If we treat learners as partners in their learning, they are more likely to treat patients as partners in their care. Because patients who work actively at taking care of themselves tend to have better health outcomes than passive patients, such an approach is highly desirable (Iverson & Vernon, 1990).

Students who were asked to assess their own performance during a clerkship in family medicine reported that they felt a sense of partnership, of "being on the same side" as their teachers. One student remarked, "Grading my own charts was a real eye-opener. I realized for the first time what my tutor had to deal with." The teachers in this clerkship said that they felt very positive about students identifying their weaknesses instead of hiding them (Henbest & Fehrsen, 1985).

To be competent and to continue learning throughout their careers, health professionals need to be reflective practitioners. Learning to provide high-quality health care is a career-long challenge. During their initial professional education, most practitioners learn about classic ways in which patients present and respond to treatment. They are also given true-false and multiple-choice exams that can cause some learners to feel that there are clear-cut "right" answers in health care. However, few patients fit neatly into classic models, and the care of patients is riddled with exceptions, uncertainties, and disagreements, so practitioners can't be satisfied with the information they memorized during their formal education. Competent patient care requires looking freshly at patients' situations, reflecting on what is and isn't working, and seeking other options, if necessary.

The array of knowledge and capabilities needed by practitioners is constantly changing and expanding. To grow throughout their careers, practitioners need to be able to learn from their experiences with patients, family members, colleagues, and others. They need to be willing and able to reflect on what they are thinking and doing, be open to new ways of functioning, be disposed to going through the discomfort of making changes, and be inclined toward monitoring their progress when making changes.

Reflective practitioners are likely to provide better patient care. In busy patient-care situations, it is natural for practitioners to develop routine ways of functioning. Some reflexive responses are efficient and help learners and practitioners function under stressful conditions. If practitioners are routinely on autopilot, however, there is a risk that they will miss important information, categorize patients incorrectly, be insufficiently empathic, and make inappropriate decisions.

Health professionals who are not reflective, self-directed, self-critical learners can become incompetent, even dangerous. After completing their formal education, many physicians and other health professionals are evaluated only rarely, and this evaluation seldom includes being observed in action. Even during their formal education, few of the examinations they take—not even certification exams—adequately evaluate their full range of capabilities as providers of patient care.

Health professionals are expected to participate in continuing education. Most of the programs that are offered, however, are didactic courses, involving little if any meaningful practice experiences or evaluation. Although health professionals are expected to monitor their own work and keep up in their field, they are typically given little help in preparing to do so. Many of us worry about the capacity of at least some of our graduates to remain competent and safe. Recent reports, such as the one by the Institute of

Medicine (Kohn, Corrigan & Donaldson, 2000), indicate that we have reason to be concerned. Earlier, Sackett and colleagues (1977) examined the competence and safety of physicians and concluded the following:

> There is growing evidence that our effectiveness as clinicians, at least in some domains, begins to deteriorate as soon as we complete our clinical training. . . . Our factual knowledge of human biology deteriorates, both because we forget it and because we fail to learn new facts as they emerge. . . . We fail to keep abreast of advances in diagnosis and therapy, and often continue to use the old (and sometimes ineffective) treatments we learned as trainees, instead of newer, more effective ones. (p. 245)

To support their contention, Sackett and colleagues cited their own study of 80 family physicians who were presented with patients with hypertension. They found that the best predictor of the physicians' approach was the year of their graduation from medical school. The longer ago they graduated, the less likely physicians were to provide appropriate treatment. (Evans et al. (1984) presented similar findings.)

Sackett, Haynes, and Tugwell (1985) concluded:

> It appears that clinicians in our part of the world continue to make the same treatment decisions they learned from their teachers, and tend not to alter these decisions after they complete their training, even when subsequent evidence dictates that they should. Thus, although they may have been taught the best medical practice available at the time of their formal education, they apparently had not been taught how to decide when their medical practice became outdated and needed to be changed. (p. 246)

Key to our graduates' continued effectiveness is ensuring that they are sufficiently committed to reflection and competent at it, so they will regularly determine when their current diagnostic and management strategies are not adequate and need to be changed. Of course, this requires that they stay up-to-date on the literature, including evidence for the effectiveness or ineffectiveness of long-standing as well as new treatments.

IN CONCLUSION

Helping students, residents, and practitioners in the health professions to become reflective practitioners is one of our key responsibilities. In this chapter we presented some of our reasons for contending that the capacity to be critically self-reflective is vital for providing high-quality patient care and for ensuring the continuing growth of practitioners. Later in this book we suggest some steps for helping learners become and remain reflective practitioners.

CHAPTER 2

Why Is Constructive Feedback Important?

Feedback is central to learning. As children, feedback from our parents and others was vital in learning verbal and nonverbal communication skills. Those of us who try learning a new language as adults also need feedback about our pronunciation, our choice of words, and our grammar. Timely, accurate, specific feedback, offered constructively, is similarly essential for becoming and remaining an effective health professional. We particularly need the reflections and feedback of others when first learning new skills, when trying to make changes in long-established ways of functioning, and when struggling with difficult patient-care challenges.

Among educators feedback is commonly defined as information that students are given about their performance with the intention of guiding them in acquiring desired attitudes and skills. Feedback can be simply descriptive or it can include some assessment, even some judgment.

For us, feedback also includes reflections on the context in which the learner is working. For instance, if a teacher is watching a student start an IV, in addition to giving the student feedback about how he did the procedure, the teacher might also share her reflections about the way the patient was reacting, the configuration of the workplace, and other factors that were linked to—and may have had an impact on—what the student was doing.

Fostering reflection and providing feedback shouldn't be separate monologues; the first delivered by the learner and the second by the teacher. Rather they should be linked components of an ongoing dialogue that we describe later. First we look at some of the reasons why constructive feedback is so essential to learning.

We cannot see ourselves as others see us.   Except for glimpses in mirrors or viewings of video recordings of ourselves, most of us don't see ourselves as others see us. In fact, when first viewing videos of ourselves, many of us are surprised by the sound of our voice, the expressions on our face, or our mannerisms. Even when watching videos of our interactions with others, we can't know fully how they or others perceive us. To know how we are perceived, we need feedback.

Reflective students and practitioners can learn to recognize clues about their impact and how they appear to others, but on their own they can only form hypotheses about these matters. Studying video recordings of their interactions with real or simulated patients can give learners a sense of how they appear to others, so we strongly recommend doing this. These recordings, however, can't present the patients' important internal experiences. Therefore, when possible, learners can benefit from patients' feedback (see Chapter 8). They can also benefit from the perceptions of teachers and other knowledgeable people who observe them in action.

Even world-class athletes and artistic performers who are skilled at self-assessment know they need the perceptions and reflections of coaches or directors. Most of these advisors are actually less skilled as performers than their students. The good ones, however, understand what is needed for excellent performance and the steps involved in getting there. The best coaches also have an understanding of human nature and behavior, enabling them to convey their reflections and feedback in a supportive, constructive way that is matched to their student's readiness.

Our perceptions are selective, and each of us can interpret the same event differently.   How we perceive the world differs from person to person. What catches our attention, what we avoid, and what we fail to see depend on such factors as our previous experiences with similar events, our understanding of what is happening, our values, biases, and level of alertness. As Anais Nin observed in her published diary, "We don't see things as they are, we see things as we are (1969)." If we are involved in an event, our perceptions are affected by such factors as what we are doing, our level of comfort with what we are doing, and what we can see as well as perceive.

A preceptor who is watching a student suture a laceration on the badly bruised arm of a young child might notice that the child shows no visible emotion and her mother appears to be very nervous. The student, who is just learning to suture and is heavily focused on doing it correctly, may not notice the child's flat affect or the mother's tension. Even if the student studies the faces of the child and mother, if he is not tuned into psychological issues, he and his preceptor might describe and interpret what they see differently. Such learners can benefit from the observations of others who see things that they don't see or interpret the same things differently, or both.

Beginners aren't equipped to give themselves feedback. When acquiring new capabilities, beginners don't know enough to assess their own performance completely or accurately. Athletes who are in the early stages of learning a skill often can't make much improvement in their performance by watching videotapes of their efforts by themselves. They need a coach to draw their attention to the key elements of performance competency (Franks & Maile, 1991). To be effective at self-critique, learners need to be sufficiently knowledgeable about the skill that they are critiquing in order to make informed judgments about what they need to change. Put another way, beginners are *unconsciously incompetent.* They know little or nothing about the new skill they are trying to learn. They don't yet have the internalized standards against which to compare their performance, and they don't know what it is they don't know. A student who doesn't yet know what open-ended questions are will not be able to perceive *if* she has used them in an interview, let alone critique *how* she has used them. Beginners need the feedback of teachers to help them recognize what they are doing and to help them critique their progress.

Over time, in a constructive learning environment, learners become conscious of what they need to be able to do, even though they have not yet mastered the new capability. They are now *consciously incompetent.* They know what they are not yet able to do, so they can begin critiquing their efforts, at least in general terms. (Subtle perceptions and refined critique require a considerably higher level of achievement.)

If all goes well, learners continue to be conscious of what is involved in doing the skills they are trying to learn, and they become reasonably accomplished at using them. They move toward being *consciously competent*. Later, after repeated use of the skill, learners may become *unconsciously competent,* a condition that has its advantages and risks. They can now perform fairly automatically, no longer needing to focus intently on what they are doing. This means they can focus on other matters simultaneously. A student who has learned to do a thorough neurological examination no longer needs to think through each step in the process. She now has the residual capacity to be critically reflective about her work while doing it. If, however, she has not been receiving constructive feedback and helped to develop the habit of being reflective, she is at risk for a diminishing capacity to continue learning through her ongoing use of that skill. Using the skill reflexively or mindlessly may work in some routine situations, but an automatic approach is likely to be inadequate for managing nonstandard circumstances. Also, if she loses touch with the steps involved in learning and perfecting that skill, she will be less able to help others learn it.

Even when they are consciously or unconsciously competent, learners need feedback from others. And with the rapid change and growth of new knowledge and skills in health care, practitioners may also become unconsciously incompetent beginners over and over again as they face the need to change or to replace established practices. In other words, health professionals need external feedback throughout their careers.

Without feedback, learning can be delayed, inefficient, or unsuccessful. Imagine trying to pick out a tune on the piano without hearing the notes you are playing, or hitting drives on a golf course without knowing where the ball lands in relation to your target. In either case, without feedback on your actions, how will you know what adjustments to make to improve your piano-playing or your golf shot?

Nearly a century ago, Thorndike (1912) reported a simple, informative experiment that demonstrated the need for specific, accurate feedback when learning. He asked people in three groups to draw lines of specific lengths freehand. One group received no feedback. They were told only to keep practicing. The second group received incomplete feedback. They were told whether their lines were too long or too short, but not by how much. The third group received specific information about how their lines differed from the assigned length. Not surprisingly to anyone who has reflected on the importance of feedback, the first group never improved. The second group improved steadily but quite slowly, never achieving consistent accuracy. In relatively few tries, however, the third group achieved striking precision in their freehand drawings.

Effective feedback can accelerate and facilitate learning.
Centuries ago, squires training to be knights learned jousting skills with an early teaching machine—a wooden figure of a knight on a pivot, holding a shield in one hand and a club in the other. The squire on horseback charged at the figure with his jousting lance poised. If he hit the shield squarely in the middle, the figure fell over. If he hit the shield off-center he received prompt negative feedback in the form of a blow from the club held by the now spinning wooden knight. Learning apparently took place quickly with this somewhat crude feedback mechanism (Angrist,1973).

Getting clubbed is hardly an optimal way to receive feedback. Feedback, however, is essential in most learning endeavors. Scheidt and colleagues (1986) demonstrated that students who received critiques from their preceptors of their videotaped patient encounters performed significantly better on the second recorded interview and examination than those who did self-guided critiques or those in the control group who received no critiques. Wigton, Kashinath, and Hoellerich (1986) reported that students who are given information about *how* they appear to use information when making judgments learn to make judgments more accurately than those who are not given this information.

Most of us want, even demand, feedback in some situations.
Although most of us have suffered from hurtful or negative feedback, we still want feedback in certain situations. If, for example, your tennis serve is off and you seek coaching, you would probably feel cheated if that coach didn't observe you and give you prompt feedback about what you needed to change. Can you imagine learning to fly an airplane without an instructor who gives you immediate feedback?

Constructive feedback ranked second only to clinical competence among family practice residents who were surveyed about their perceptions of the elements of effective teaching (Wolverton & Bosworth, 1985). In another study, medical students who were learning clinical skills preferred receiving feedback during, rather than after, going through OSCEs (objective structured clinical examinations) (Black & Harden, 1986). In yet another study, medical residents who interviewed a standardized patient were asked to decide whether they wanted feedback from others. Ninety percent (90%) chose to review a video recording of their patient interview with a preceptor who provides feedback; 60% chose to do their reviews with peers and patients included (O'Sullivan, Pinsker, & Landou, 1991).

Without feedback, mistakes remain uncorrected and bad habits can develop. As we've noted, practice does not automatically make perfect. It is not uncommon for advanced students and residents to do procedures or parts of patient exams incorrectly and not know it. Some have never been observed or have not been given the feedback they needed to recognize and correct their errors.

Years ago as a consultant to a national medical specialty certification board, one of us (HJ) observed multiple candidates as they did their required physical exams of assigned patients. He saw a good number of candidates commit a variety of errors. Like most students and residents who perform incorrectly, these candidates didn't realize they were doing anything wrong. Not having witnessed these workups, their assigned examiners had no way of knowing about the errors. After doing their patient workups, the candidates went to another room where they reported their findings to their examiners. Understandably, no one reported such observations as, "I palpated in the wrong place when checking for thyroid enlargement," even though several of them had actually done so. They reported what they believed: that their patients' thyroids were not enlarged, which in all cases happened to be correct. Neither they nor their examiners realized that they had done that and other parts of the physical exam incorrectly. If the *information* or conclusion a learner provides is correct we should not assume that the *process* used to acquire that information or arrive at that conclusion was necessarily correct.

Without feedback, learners may drop desirable behaviors.
As suspected by some teachers and confirmed several decades ago by Eron (1955) and Helfer (1970), the attitudes and capabilities of some students deteriorate during their medical education. If learners

are not helped to recognize their strengths, they are at risk of discontinuing desirable behaviors. Beginners, for example, who are inherently sensitive to patients' concerns, or who instinctively adopt an open-ended approach to interviewing, may not know they have these capabilities or that these approaches are valued. They need reinforcing feedback.

Many of the students and residents with whom we have talked during hundreds of workshops and consultations report that they seldom receive positive feedback. Glenn, Reid, Mahaffy, and Shurtleff (1984) found this to be true in their study of 949 separate consultations between residents and attending physicians in two ambulatory care centers. Only 3.4% of these consultations included positive feedback (some form of reinforcement or praise).

Without feedback, learners may make inaccurate assumptions. When needed or expected feedback is missing, some learners conclude they are not doing well even though they may be. Other learners assume they are doing well when, in fact, their performance is inadequate. The minimal amount of helpful feedback learners receive in most schools causes many of them to be constantly vigilant for evidence of feedback from their teachers. When explicit feedback is not forthcoming, learners are inclined to fill the vacuum with whatever crumbs are available and with their own assumption.

Inaccurate or incomplete feedback is not helpful to learning. A student who observes that her preceptor looks discouraged and unhappy may conclude that the preceptor is dissatisfied with something she did. The preceptor, however, may look that way because one of his patients just had an unexpected setback. He may actually be satisfied with the student's work.

When feedback is insufficient, the importance of formal tests can be inflated. Most written tests and other formal evaluations measure only a small, often minimally important part of what future health professionals need. As well summarized a while ago in a report by the panel on the General Professional Education of the Physician (GPEP, 1984), "Examinations cannot replace reasoned, analytical, personal evaluations of the specific skills and overall abilities of students" (p. 13).

The episodic, superficial, and incomplete information provided by most formal testing gives our learners and us only partial, static snapshots of the complex, changing landscape of their intellectual and performance skills. Instead, they and we need the far richer information that can derive from day-to-day observation. If test scores and occasional comments are the learners' primary or only sources of feedback, they are likely to attribute far more weight to these sources than they deserve. In their determination to survive their professional education, some students put far more effort into preparing for these exams than into developing their clinical skills, judgment, sensitivity, or other attributes needed for optimal functioning as professionals. In such educational environments, some students are distracted from their goal of becoming effective practitioners, rather than helped to move closer to it.

IN CONCLUSION

The central importance of accurate, timely, frequent feedback in learning is not a new revelation. Yet constructive feedback remains relatively rare in health professions education. In this chapter we summarized some of the primary reasons why effective feedback is vital to optimal learning and patient care. Next we review some of the reasons why this essential educational component is often missing and, by implication, what we can do to change this situation.

CHAPTER 3

Why Are Reflection and Feedback Avoided or Done Poorly?

There is growing recognition of the importance of fostering the development of reflective practitioners (Boud, Keogh, & Walkers, 1985; Epstein, 1999; Johns & Freshwater, 1998; Mezirow, 1998; Papell & Skolnik, 1992; Schön, 1987). Some attention has been given to reflecting on experiences, particularly in the learning of interpersonal skills (e.g., Brock & Stock, 1990; DeTornyay & Thompson, 1982; Jason et al., 1971; Kahn et al., 1979; Westberg et al., 1980). However, in general, relatively little attention is given to this process in health professions curricula.

Particularly in the early years of their formal education, too many students spend considerable time passively listening to lectures and trying to cram facts into their heads so they can pass exams. Such activities not only fail to provide experiences that are worthy of reflection, they can work against the development of the habits of mind needed for being appropriately reflective. Even in those programs that provide learners with worthy experiences, the pressure to run from one experience to the next with little or no time for basic physiological functions, let alone reflection, often diminishes learners' opportunities to be reflective. It is not uncommon for learners to forget important aspects of these rushed experiences. In addition, learners typically get insufficient exposure to reflective role models and little guidance in how to be reflective.

Timely, accurate, specific feedback, delivered constructively, is also vital for learning. Yet in many schools of the health professions, students don't get adequate feedback (Irby, 1995; Isaacson, Posk, Litaker, & Halperin, 1995; Remmen et al., 2000). Irby (1986) reported that students at the University of Washington School of Medicine who rated the clinical teaching at their institution gave teachers the lowest score in "provides direction and feedback." Irby said this is not unique to his institution and that feedback from written evaluations of students' performance is as inadequate as oral feedback because of faculty members' lack of specificity in identifying students' strengths and weaknesses.

When faculty members think they are providing feedback, their students do not always agree (Lye, Bragg, & Simpson,1997). Collins, Cassie, and Daggett (1978) found that 79% of the physician faculty members they surveyed felt they were assessing their trainees' skills on rounds. Only 46% of the trainees perceived that such assessments were occurring. Similarly, Stritter, Haines, and Grimes (1975) found that groups of teachers consistently asserted they provided far more and better feedback than their students felt they received.

Typically, health professions teachers provide feedback at the end of courses or clinical learning experiences when it is too late for learners to use the information in that experience. Much as pilots need a continuing stream of information so they can make appropriate midcourse corrections, learners need to be kept constantly aware of where they are in relation to their learning goals (their destinations), if they are to make steady progress. Further, much of what is provided (grades, general summaries, casual comments) is insufficiently descriptive or precise to be useful.

Why are reflection and feedback typically avoided or done poorly in the health professions? That's our focus in this chapter.

Many educators have had few models of reflection or constructive feedback to emulate. During our work with thousands of health professions teachers, we've asked about their experiences with reflection and feedback during their own education. Most report receiving little or no encouragement or time for reflection and say that they were rarely asked to critique their own work. Most also said that they received no guidance in how to assess their work. Many report that as students they received little or no truly constructive feedback and that the limited amount of feedback they received was often unpleasant, poorly timed, insensitive, not based on direct knowledge of their work, and even hurtful.

Fostering reflection and providing constructive feedback are complex skills. Helping learners become reflective practitioners and providing them with useful feedback are challenging tasks for which most health professions educators have had little or no preparation (Jason & Westberg, 1982). These are primarily human process skills, so guidelines and rules alone are insufficient. Most of us need considerable practice developing and refining these skills, and we need feedback on our efforts.

Teachers and learners avoid negative feedback. Most of us are uncomfortable being the bearer of bad news. Ende (1983) says that when teachers are committed to the importance of feedback but uneasy about the impact it will have on learners, they tend to talk around the learner's problems, use indirect statements, or speak in generalities and abstractions, essentially obfuscating their messages. The following are some examples of what he calls vanishing feedback: "For your level of training, you did fine." "You seem to be making satisfactory progress." "You were clearly trying during your time on this service." Such observations convey nothing that contributes to the learner's growth.

In turn, many learners fear that any effort they might make to elicit more meaningful feedback may bring a negative evaluation. They support and reinforce the teacher's avoidance of what should be a central issue between them. The result, despite the best of intentions, is that nothing of any real value gets transmitted or received.

Certainly we take a risk when we give negative feedback to learners. We are opening the possibility that the recipient of our feedback will become angry and might even retaliate in some way. Or we may worry that we will cause so much distress we will interfere with the learner's development. However, as we describe later, if our feedback is presented constructively and we convey our genuine desire to be helpful, negative feedback can actually deepen, not diminish, our relationships with learners. In addition their learning is likely to be enhanced.

Teachers who received hurtful feedback as students are at risk of providing feedback in hurtful ways. Few if any teachers intend to be hurtful to learners. Yet even without intending to, teachers who have been the recipients of hurtful feedback are at risk of treating others similarly. A well-recognized, tragic illustration of this phenomenon is the perpetuation of child abuse. A high proportion of parents who abuse children were themselves abused as children (Helfer & Kempe, 1976). Teachers who don't have positive models to emulate are at risk of replicating their own experiences when they give feedback to their students, unless they work hard to ensure that they break the cycle.

McKegney (1989) drew disturbing parallels between some of what happens in medical education and in neglectful, abusive family systems:

> Negative judgment is common at all levels of medical education; direct feedback, which cites specifics and offers suggestions for improvement, is rare. Like adults who were scolded more than they were instructed as children, physicians have difficulty discerning the differences between describing behavior and labeling the person "good" or "bad." Because clear feedback is rare and correction is more common than affirmation, the medical trainee has difficulty feeling competent. Receiving punishing comments about mistakes teaches trainees to hide errors, by lying if necessary. Like emotionally abused children, residents become unwilling to risk the pain they have come to associate with close observation and eventually learn to avoid supervision. The absence of honest, constructive feedback and the overabundance of placing blame in medical education perpetuate physicians' perfectionism and leave them at risk for impairment (p. 454).

Competitive environments make self-disclosure risky. Getting accepted into and making progress in schools in the health professions can be highly competitive processes. Many students are in a noncollaborative mode well before they enter these programs. Competition often continues in residencies and other graduate programs

Most of us want to look good to the world and so try to shut out information that runs counter to our desired image (Porter, 1982). In competitive environments with an abundance of perfectionists, learners tend to try to hide rather than disclose anything about themselves that they worry may be perceived as deficiencies. Even if we are trying to create environments in which deficiencies are not held against learners, we may need to make special efforts to convince learners that it is safe for them to be open with us.

In large-group teaching, gathering essential information about learner performance is difficult. The more we're able to directly observe learners using the skills they need for patient care, the more we can foster reflection and provide accurate, meaningful feedback. Large-group teaching, which is the norm during the early years of most professional education, provides little opportunity for learners to practice relevant skills, let alone for teachers to observe them doing so. This limitation is especially true when teachers present traditional lectures in which they talk *at* learners rather than interact *with* or listen *to* them.

Some teachers engage learners in activities that provide glimpses of skills that are relevant to patient care. For example, a teacher might ask a student to think aloud about how she would work through a clinical challenge. However, in the typical 50-minute large group session, there rarely is time for teachers to watch most learners in action.

Educators who work with large groups of learners usually gather most of their information about learners through written examinations. Well-designed exams can provide some helpful information, such as how learners think through problems. The information gathered from many traditional exams, however, provides an incomplete, even distorted picture of the learners' full range of capabilities, especially those that are central to being effective practicing professionals.

Many schools in the health professions are reducing the amount of time devoted to large group teaching and increasing the amount of time that learners spend in small groups. Small groups in which learners reflect aloud on their patient care experiences, jointly work on solving clinical problems, or practice clinical exam skills with each other give small group facilitators some access to learners' capabilities, making it possible for the facilitators to encourage reflection and provide useful feedback (Westberg & Jason, 1996).

Finding time for reflection and feedback in crowded curricula or in busy clinical settings can be difficult. With the growing knowledge base in the health sciences, most faculty members already feel that important topics are being left out of the curriculum. Teachers and departments compete for more curriculum time and worry that they can't do all they consider important within the time they've been allotted. In this atmosphere, proposals to set aside time for reflection and feedback tend to be dismissed. In the clinical setting, administrators push practitioners to see more and more patients each day, so requests to protect time for reflection and feedback also can be rejected unless strong arguments are mounted.

Until a reflective mind-set is well established, extra time and effort are required. To be reflective, learners often need reminders from others. Once reflection is habitual, learners tend to be reflective at times when they would be daydreaming or otherwise passing time between events.

Productivity is valued more highly than reflection. The problem of finding time for reflection and feedback is exacerbated by the fact that, like the outside world, the cultures of most health professions schools and health care settings put a high premium on being busy and productive. Workaholism is rampant and has permeated medicine for decades. "Good" students and practitioners are expected to work long hours, even when this can be harmful to their health and to their family life. Gordon (1999) says that taking time to reflect is counter to the dominant culture and that it might be more difficult for faculty than for students to change the culture.

IN CONCLUSION

Given the ways many teachers were treated as learners and the economic and time pressures that dominate many educational settings, it's not surprising that reflection and feedback are not adequately provided for in most programs. We hope that the arguments for including them (see Chapters 1 and 2) will help convince you that it is worth making every effort to do so in your program. In the chapters ahead we offer steps and strategies for increasing the presence and enhancing the quality of these instructional components in programs in which you participate.

CHAPTER 4

Preparing Yourself
and Your Learners

Given the limited and often inadequate experiences many teachers and learners have had with reflection and feedback, special preparation is often needed for these processes to go well. At faculty development workshops and seminars we ask teachers to identify challenges they have faced or anticipate facing when helping learners reflect on and assess their work or when providing feedback to learners. Common concerns include how to deal with learners who would rather be "doing" than reflecting and learners who are defensive, insufficiently self-aware, or overly self-critical. Teachers also wonder what to do when learners ignore or discount their feedback or reject them for being the bearers of bad news.

These and other challenges are often best addressed directly, as early as possible, or by preventing them from happening in the first place. The following are some steps to consider taking before inviting learners to reflect aloud on their work or before giving them feedback.

PREPARING YOURSELF

Reflect on your experiences with and attitudes toward reflection, including self-assessment. Our own experiences can be a rich resource for our work. However, since we may inadvertently treat others in ways that we were treated, we need to be fully aware of both our positive and negative prior experiences. Some

questions to consider: During your own education, were you encouraged to be reflective? If so, did you learn any lessons about the
reflection process and about self-assessment that you'd like to use in
your teaching? Do you now take time to reflect on (and critique)
your work as an educator or practitioner? If so, how helpful are
these steps in your ongoing learning? If you aren't habitually reflective, what might be getting in the way?

Reflect on your experiences with receiving feedback.   Reflect
on experiences that were helpful to you and those you found
unpleasant, even hurtful. Try to remember experiences you've had
not only in your professional education, but also in sports or the arts
outside school. What were some of the ingredients of those experiences that were helpful to you? Who provided the feedback? How
was it conveyed? Did you have hurtful experiences that you want to
be sure not to repeat with your learners?

Reflect on your experiences with giving feedback.   Think of
times when you provided feedback in effective, constructive ways.
What did you do that you want to be sure to do routinely when providing feedback in the future? Reflect also on times when you feel
you provided feedback ineffectively. Can you identify any conditions
in the setting or in your own disposition at the time that may have
contributed to your being less effective than you would have wished?
Did you learn any lessons that you want to bring to the feedback you
will be offering from now on?

Make certain that you are clear about the learning goals.
During courses and clinical experiences, health professions students are—or should be—expected to develop or enhance some
specific knowledge, attitudes, and/or skills. When they finish the
course they should be able to do things that they weren't able to do
when they began. If the course director or others expect you to guide
learners in achieving certain learning goals, you need to know what
these goals are. When educators are asked to teach a course or
supervise learners, too often they are given only a vague notion of
what they are expected to work on with the learners.

   The capabilities that learners are expected to develop should be
described in advance, in writing. These goals should be worthy,
clearly stated, appropriate for the learners' stage of development,

and achievable within the time and resources available (Westberg & Jason, 1993). Ideally, you and others who are working directly with the students will be involved in formulating these learning goals.

If you are not a clinician, we encourage you to be clear about the link between what you are expected to teach and what your learners will need to do as practitioners. If you are uncertain, consider talking with clinicians and even spending time in a clinical setting.

In addition to these preestablished goals, learners should be encouraged to formulate their own learning goals. In fact, on some electives there are no preestablished goals and learners are expected to develop their own. (We discuss learner-generated goals in the next chapter.)

Provide opportunities for learners to practice what they need to learn. The health professions are performing arts. As we described earlier, practitioners need to be able to do such things as elicit and provide information, identify and solve problems, collect and critically review needed information, and communicate effectively with patients and families. In clinical settings students and residents have opportunities to do these things, although if they are working on particular skills you might need to arrange specific experiences for them. Even in the classroom though, students can practice the skills they'll need. For example, if you're working with them on communication skills, you can ask them to practice with each other or with standardized patients. (Standardized patients are people who have been trained to present as patients with certain stories and symptoms.) If you are a scientist and are trying to help learners understand how the body functions and how to be problem solvers, you can build the learning around patient care situations and exercises that give learners practice in gathering scientific information and in identifying and solving problems.

Try to observe your learners using the capabilities they are expected to develop while working with you. You and the learners can reflect together on experiences they've had that you haven't witnessed. To be maximally helpful, however, actually observe them in action, at least occasionally. Directly observing learners can give you a clearer sense of their capabilities and areas of need. You might also observe some important things that they failed to perceive or didn't think to bring to your attention. With the primary data of direct observation, you are likely to be better equipped to help learners reflect on how to improve their skills.

If you are supervising learners in clinical settings, consider observing learners directly or on video as they work with patients. If you are working with students in the community, consider joining them occasionally as they work with members of the community. If you are facilitating a small group of learners, perhaps you can observe them as they work with their peers in trying to solve problems, raise questions of you and their peers, and offer their opinions about a topic under discussion.

If your only access to learners will be in large groups, you may not have adequate exposure to most of them. Consider dividing the learners into small groups at times and have them engage in problem solving, role-playing, or other activities where they simulate what they will be doing in the real world. As the groups meet, you can circulate among them and observe them. You can also ask learners to write papers and respond to exams. Unless you design your tests with considerable care, however, you may be learning more about how skilled they are at taking tests than how well they think or do other tasks that are relevant to their future.

Whether you will be working with large or small groups or with individuals, you might want to plan to take notes on your observations while they are fresh in your mind. As in patient care, our memory for details can fade quickly, and, as we discuss later, details are essential in order to be optimally helpful to learners.

Find ways to include the learners' reflection and your feedback in your work together.   When learners engage in classroom experiences, like those described above, you can include time for them to reflect on what they did. For example, after a group of students or residents has jointly worked through a paper-based clinical problem, you can ask them to individually write down their reflections about how they functioned in this team process and then share their reflections with all of you. Next the students can offer feedback to each other, and you can give them feedback on their process. (In Chapter 7 we discuss ways for peers to reflect with and give feedback to one another.)

If you will be teaching in a clinical setting, reflection-in-action can be built around the learners' interactions with patients and other clinical activities. The long tradition of teaching at the bedside in the presence of the patient has rich possibilities for reflection and feedback, if done with sufficient sensitivity to the needs and feelings of the patient and student. Reflection and feedback can also take place in the presence of ambulatory patients. While learners are performing certain exams and procedures, you can engage them in reflecting aloud about their thinking and actions, and you can provide feedback as needed. If the student will be doing a procedure where an error could be painful or harmful to the patient, you can ask the student to do anticipatory thinking aloud, telling you what she intends to do at each key step but then stopping and inviting your feedback before proceeding.

If you expect that the student will have already done a patient workup and may even have a management plan before you come into the exam room, you can ask the student to reflect aloud on his or her thinking in the patient's presence. Then you can provide constructive feedback, even corrective feedback as needed. (In Chapters 5 and 8, we discuss ways of doing this that are helpful to students and not hurtful to patients.)

Arseneau (1995) points out that in the hospital students do not have time for much reflection during intake and attending rounds. He recommends holding exit rounds during which patient care situations can be discussed in their entirety.

Identify private, quiet locations for talking with learners. Some reflection and feedback can be done in front of others. However, conversations that learners perceive as personal, as touching on their basic capabilities or personalities, or as having potentially negative consequences for their evaluations should take place in protected settings, such as a private office where you can close the door. There are exceptions. If you are working with a small group of learners who trust one another, you can provide some sensitive individual feedback in the presence of the group, particularly if you are offering constructive advice and if the others can learn from your exchanges with individuals. Regardless of where or with whom you have these conversations, try to find a quiet place.

Many clinicians find it best to put these supervisory sessions on their clinical appointment schedule so the time is protected. When left to chance, supervisory sessions are often preempted by the inevitable arrival of other pressing tasks.

Find out what roles if any, you and your learners have in evaluating their work.   If you will be making judgments about learners that will be part of their permanent record, they are likely to be guarded about what they disclose to you regarding their areas of concern or need. But they might be more forthcoming if they are convinced that you really want to help them and that you need to know their problem areas and deficiencies to do so. Earning this level of trust from learners is probably our highest achievement as teachers and usually requires careful advance thought, preparation, and well-developed personal skill. (Earning learners' trust is just as important for teachers as earning patients' trust is for clinicians.)

Consider eliciting feedback about the learners' work from others.   Other members of the health team can offer unique perspectives on the learners' work. For example, physicians and social workers can provide useful observations to nursing students. Nurses can provide useful critique to medical students and residents (Butterfield, Mazzaferri, & Sachs, 1987; Linn, Oye, Cope, & DiMatteo, 1986; McCue, Marginat, Hansen, & Bailey, 1986; Norcini, Shea, & Webster, 1986; Shatney & Friend, 1984).

If you plan to elicit feedback for your learners from other health professionals, ensure that the other professionals are only asked for feedback in areas in which they have expertise and relevant information. For example, it would be inappropriate to ask most physicians to comment about a nursing student's skills in making a nursing diagnosis. It might be appropriate though to ask physicians about a nursing student's functioning as a member of the health team.

In a growing number of schools, students spend time learning and working in communities. In some schools, community leaders and other members of the community who have significant involvement with students participate in evaluating the students' work (Kaufman, 1985; Schmidt, Magzoub, Feletti, Nooman, & Vluggen, 2000). Later, we discuss eliciting feedback from standardized and real patients and from other students.

Identify or create forms that can facilitate reflection and feedback.   To help guide the learners' reflections, consider creating a form with questions for the learners to respond to after selected experiences. If you have many questions for the learners' reflection, consider creating a checklist. For example, a checklist that learners could use after doing a procedure on a patient might include the following items: Did I explain to the patient what I was going to do? Did I give the patient an opportunity to ask questions? Were there any surprises during the session? If so, how did I deal with them?

To encourage learners to assess what they did in more depth, you might use an assessment form linked to the attitudes, skills, and other capabilities that the learners are expected to develop. Parallel forms—those in which the same items appear on the forms used by the teacher and the student—can be especially helpful. For example, both forms might include an item pertaining to the student's capacity to listen actively to patients. If you and the student each complete the assessment form independently and then share what you wrote, the student can compare his self-assessment with yours. This provides the student with feedback on his self-assessment.

Items that appear on the learners' assessment forms can also appear on assessment forms used by peers, other health professionals, patients, and community leaders. These groups should be asked to provide feedback only on items about which they are qualified to comment, and a plan is needed to ensure that the learners get this feedback in a timely way. Be certain that the content of that feedback and the way it is conveyed are helpful.

Note: If you have told the learners that the information on the forms is to be used only as feedback, then you must make sure that the completed forms are not used for grading.

Consider using videotape recordings of the learners' work.
A powerful strategy for facilitating reflection and providing feedback is videotaping learners as they practice tasks, such as interacting with patients. Sports coaches have long recognized the usefulness of having athletes review recordings of practice sessions and games (McCallum, 1987). We are among those educators in the health professions who have found video to be very valuable, and we enthusiastically urge its wider use (Westberg & Jason, 1994b).

There are numerous arguments for using video recordings. First, you don't have to be present during the actual event, such as your student's encounter with a patient. Video recordings enable learners to have some sense of how others see them. Learners are far more likely to gain value from watching themselves than by having someone else try to describe what they did. Video provides you and learners with an objective record of what happened, so you don't have to spend time trying to recall details, and you can avoid wasteful disputes that arise when you and they have different recollections of the same event.

Watching themselves on video can even help learners recall what they were thinking and feeling at the time. If they choose, they can replay sections of the interaction, focusing each time on a separate component. They can also stop at key decision points, such as after a statement or other action by the patient. They can then reflect on what they did or said, and they can think through various options that were available at the time, enriching their repertoire for future encounters.

Most schools and programs now have video equipment that can be used for taping learners as they interact with patients. If your school or program doesn't have the equipment, consider using an inexpensive home camcorder.

Consider using literature to foster reflective practice. Some educators advocate inviting learners and health professionals to read and reflect on patient narratives, short stories, poems, and excerpts from novels that describe the experience of illness, the experience of caring for people, and the relationship between patients and health professionals. Reading and reflecting on this literature, they say, allows learners to enter the intimate world of other health professionals and patients, enabling learners to better appreciate the perspectives of others, to be more empathic with their own patients, to have a greater understanding of their own feelings, and to be aware of alternative responses to challenging situations (Charon, et al., 1995; Shapiro & Lie, 2000). After learners read literature that presents the experience of patients, you can stimulate discussions with questions like "How does the world look from the patient's perspective?" and "What might explain the patient's behavior?" (Shapiro & Lie, 2000). Discussions of this sort may remind learners of their own patients and cause them to want to reflect again on particularly poignant or challenging situations.

Consider inviting learners to express their experience in some artistic form. Expressing experiences in an artistic form can make those experiences available for richer, subtler levels of reflection. Consider inviting learners and practitioners to recall in detail a story from their work with patients (their practice) and then to render the meaning of that story in some artful expression, such as poetry, music, sculpture, or dance. When learners express themselves artistically, they can make discoveries that are difficult to access through more conventional approaches to reflection (Schoenhofer, Personal Communication, November, 2000; Boykin & Schoenhofer, 1991, 1993). Shapiro and Lie (2000) note that "creative writing encourages a certain empathy or tenderness because it requires a willingness to enter unreservedly—if only in one's imagination—into the patient's world." They found that when residents wrote a brief poem or a couple of paragraphs about a "difficult" patient, some of them had new insights into the patients' illness experience. Some even came up with new ideas for working more effectively with this type of patient.

PREPARING LEARNERS

Most of the following steps apply when working with learners one-on-one or in groups in either classroom or clinical settings. We cannot supply examples for all situations, so please focus on the principles and strategies and think through how they might apply in the context in which you teach.

If you're going to be working one-on-one with learners, you can prepare them one at a time. If you're going to be working one-on-one with several learners, consider bringing them together in a group and preparing them at the same time. If you will be working with a group of learners who will be collectively fostering each other's learning and providing feedback, these steps—plus others that we describe in Chapter 7—can be taken in the group.

Learners vary in their experiences and comfort with reflection and feedback. If learners are new to reflection and feedback or have had negative prior experiences, be prepared to give extra effort to the following steps.

Build trust.   Our effectiveness in helping learners reflect accurately on their work and be appropriately critical depends upon our ability to first earn their trust. Learners who don't trust us are likely to withhold observations about themselves. Even if they have good insights about their needs, they will probably share their concerns with us only if they are convinced we are truly their advocates and able to help them.

Because many learners have had unpleasant, even humiliating experiences with feedback, developing this level of trust is seldom easy or quick. To earn our students' and residents' trust as early as possible in our relationships, we need to honestly feel and demonstrate that our feedback is given in the spirit of caring and concern. If we want learners to invite our feedback, we need to convince them that we are competent, credible sources of helpful feedback. This process can take time, so we need to be patient. Some of the steps described here and in later chapters can help build trust.

If you will be fostering reflection and providing feedback with a group of learners rather than one learner at a time, the task of building trust is even more complicated because you also need to build trust among all group members. (We address this issue in Chapter 7.)

Determine the learners' prior experiences, comfort with, and attitudes toward reflection, including self-assessment. In patient care, we don't begin an initial encounter with an intervention. First we gather information so we can adapt what we do and say to the patient's unique needs. Similarly, in educational encounters we need to begin by getting to know learners and their experience with and attitudes toward whatever we're planning to focus on with them. The following are some "diagnostic" questions to consider asking:

- What kinds of experiences, if any, have you had so far in systematically reflecting on your experiences with patients? [or whatever you'll be asking the learner to reflect on]
- Have you had any experience assessing your work? If so, how has it gone?
- Do you think that self-assessment does (or could) help you improve your skills? If so, why and how?

Many learners have had little or no prior practice reflecting systematically on their work and are unready to do so initially. They may need your guidance, encouragement, and patience.

Invite the learners to explore why reflection, including self-assessment, can be important and helpful to them. Some relevant arguments are presented in Chapter 1. For example, one reason that learners need to be reflective is that their ongoing competence as clinicians will rest on their capacity to be accurately self-critical.

Explore some of the roadblocks to reflection, especially self-assessment. We identified some roadblocks in Chapter 3. One potential obstacle we recommend discussing with virtually all learners who are new to self-assessment is the common fear that if they are open about their areas of confusion and need, that information will be used against them. This potential impediment may be particularly significant if you will be involved in grading them. Consequently, we recommend being candid about any part you will play in making formal judgments about their work. Conversely, let them know if the information they provide about their learning needs will be used only by you and them to enable you to jointly formulate a plan for helping them develop the capabilities they will need. If your program expects learners to become good at self-assessment and rewards them for doing it well, then learners will have added reasons for being open about their needs. If your program doesn't give direct recognition for this skill in the evaluation system, we encourage you to do what you can to help your program make the needed changes.

Consider modeling reflection, including self-assessment. A powerful way to illustrate reflection and to help convince learners of its usefulness is by doing it yourself in their presence. For example, you can discuss a difficult patient-care situation that you are facing, reflecting aloud about your thoughts and feelings. Even invite their reflections on your dilemmas. If you will be asking learners to reflect using video recordings of their interactions with patients, you can begin by reviewing with them a segment of a videotape of your interaction with a patient. If you're not a clinician, you could briefly describe how you use reflection in your work.

Talk with learners about the conditions under which it will be most comfortable for them to reflect on their experiences and hear your feedback. Acknowledge that many of us are uncomfortable critiquing our work and receiving feedback, especially negative feedback, in the presence of others, particularly teachers. Let them know that you want your dialogue to be as comfortable as possible. Ask them if they have had any particularly positive or negative experiences with self-reflection or feedback that might affect your work together.

Describe any steps that you want to take to help them be comfortable. For example, you might tell them that you will wait to have privacy before talking about sensitive issues with them. You might also say that you want them to tell you if they are feeling overloaded and want to postpone hearing your feedback. Invite the learners to think of other ways to make review sessions as comfortable as possible. (See Chapter 7 for ways of providing safety in group review sessions.)

Learners need feedback, so you can't withhold it, even if learners have been harmed by improper previous feedback. You can, however, adjust what you do to be as sensitive as possible to their needs. In addition, you can work with learners so they can become better able to receive and even request feedback. And, as we have emphasized, a systematic strategy of beginning reviews by inviting self-assessment often diminishes and sometimes eliminates the need for you to convey negative feedback.

Talk about ways to do reflection and feedback in the presence of patients.   Many of us have witnessed and heard horror stories of insensitive teaching sessions in the presence of patients. Such insensitivity has occurred at patients' bedsides, in ambulatory settings, and in classrooms and conference rooms. Too often patients are treated as objects rather than as people. Also, they may be unnecessarily frightened by statements made in their presence that they don't understand. In addition, too many teachers humiliate learners by giving them harsh, negative feedback in front of patients.

The patient's welfare must be foremost at all times. You and your learners might want to jointly devise some appropriate strategies, such as the following:

- Inform patients about the teaching that you propose and secure their consent.
- Use language that the patient understands.
- Consider ways to educate patients about their bodies and aspects of their condition while educating the learners.
- Encourage patients to let you and the learners know if you say or do anything that is confusing or disturbing.
- Save for private conversations any subjects that might be unnecessarily discomforting to patients.

In patient-care settings, also consider having a subtle signal between you and the learners to indicate that you or they want to consult privately outside the patient's room. Remember, though, that some tough issues can be discussed constructively in the presence of and with patients. In fact, if educators and learners don't discuss certain issues, some alert patients may notice this and worry that something is terribly wrong with them that you think they can't handle.

If constructive learning is to occur in the presence of the learners' patients, learners need to know that you are their ally who will support their relationship with the patient and give them constructive guidance if needed. In the next chapter we discuss some ways to do this.

IN CONCLUSION

As with effective health care, high-quality teaching involves careful preparation and considerable attention to prevention. If the many preparatory and preventive steps summarized in this chapter were not already part of your instructional approach, consider focusing on only a few at a time until they are fully part of your routine. The two checklists that follow may help serve as reminders of steps you want to take.

PREPARING MYSELF

A Self-Checklist

❑ ✔

Do I . . .

❑   reflect on my own experiences with and attitudes toward reflection, including self-assessment?

❑   reflect on my own experiences with receiving and giving feedback?

❑   make certain that I'm clear about the learning goals for the course?

❑   provide opportunities for learners to practice what they need to learn?

❑   try to observe learners as they use the capabilities they are expected to develop while working with me?

❑   find out ways to include reflection and feedback in my teaching?

❑   identify private, quiet locations for talking with learners?

❑   find out what roles, if any, the learners and I have in evaluating their work?

❑   consider eliciting feedback about the learners' work from others?

❑   identify or create forms that can facilitate reflection and feedback?

❑   consider using videotape recordings of the learners' work?

❑   consider using literature to foster reflective practice?

❑   consider inviting learners to express their experience in some artistic form?

PREPARING LEARNERS

A Self-Checklist

❑ ✔

Do I . . .

❑   build trust with learners?

❑   determine the learners' prior experiences, comfort with, and attitudes toward, reflection, including self-assessment?

❑   invite the learners to explore why reflection, including self-assessment, can be important and helpful to them?

❑   explore some of the roadblocks to reflection, especially self-assessment?

❑   consider modeling reflection, including self-assessment?

❑   talk with learners about the conditions under which it will be most comfortable for them to reflect on their experiences and hear my feedback?

❑   talk about ways to do reflection and feedback in the presence of patients?

CHAPTER 5

Fostering Reflection

I n the previous chapter we discussed ways to prepare yourself and your learners for the process of helping them be reflective about their experiences in the classroom, the community, and patient care settings. The steps we recommended included finding space, time, and tools for fostering reflection and providing feedback. We also emphasized the importance of building trust with learners, determining their experiences and attitudes toward reflection and feedback, and trying to jointly find ways to make the experience of being reflective and providing feedback as comfortable as possible for the learners.

In this chapter we focus on ways that you can foster your learners' reflections, including self-assessments. In Chapter 7 we look at ways that you can help students and residents foster each other's reflections.

Here we present a series of steps that you can consider taking with one or more learners before, during, and after a learning experience. There usually isn't time to attend to all the steps each time you work with learners, but these steps can serve as reminders of issues that you can address over an extended period of time when working with learners on multiple occasions.

As indicated, we regard reflection and feedback as part of a dialogue. Following an experience, you might first invite the learner's reflections. After trying to draw as much from the learner as possible, you might offer some feedback. Your feedback could trigger some further reflections from the learner, which might lead you to offer further feedback and so on.

BEFORE THE EXPERIENCE

Discuss any preestablished learning goals. If the course or clinical experience in which you'll be teaching has already formulated written learning goals, you can begin by reviewing them with the learners to ensure that they know what will be expected of them during your time together. If the goals include complex skills, such as measuring arterial blood gasses or giving bad news to patients, you can help the learners understand the challenges that lie ahead by offering demonstrations as a supplement to whatever discussions you have.

Most of us work hardest on goals that we value and for which we feel some ownership. If learners don't feel that some of the goals are worthy, one of your tasks may be to understand why that is so and to help them appreciate the importance of those goals, if appropriate.

Encourage learners to set their own goals. Particularly after they graduate, but even during their formal education, health professionals need to be constantly setting new learning goals for themselves based on such sources as their reflection on their work, feedback from others, their changing (growing) expectations, and their introduction to new knowledge and strategies from reading and seminars. Rather than limiting yourselves to preestablished goals, you might want to invite learners to set additional goals for themselves, in part as practice for doing something that is required of life-long, self-directed learners. If a student is doing an elective experience with you, there may not be any preestablished learning goals, so some early discussion of goals is vital for providing direction in your work together. If learners have their own goals, consider asking them to put these goals in writing, so that you and they can review them from time to time as you monitor their progress.

Usually it's not practical or even possible to address all of the course's learning goals every time that you work with learners, so, prior to explicit experiences, such as doing a problem-solving exercise in the classroom or seeing patients during an afternoon clinic, invite learners to identify one or two learning goals that they particularly want to work on during that event.

Invite learners to assess where they are starting from. To help learners develop a good plan for achieving their learning goals, you and they need to know their starting point. If you're working with a small number of learners, you can talk informally with them about their experience and level of comfort with the various skills they will be working on. If you need to assess the base-line skills of numerous students and residents, consider developing a self-assessment inventory in which you list the skills they are to develop and then ask them to indicate their level of experience and comfort with each of these skills. Giving learners a pretest can also help you and them assess their knowledge base. Regardless of how the assessment is done, assure the learners that the information they reveal will be used to guide your work together and will not be held against them or be used for grading them.

Encourage learners to have questions ready to ask themselves, or suggest some to get them started. Much of constructive reflection is the product of questions we ask ourselves while doing or witnessing a process. The more sophisticated a professional becomes, the more questions she is likely to bring to whatever she does or sees other do. Beginners may need guidance in formulating an initial set of questions to ask themselves when they engage in experiences in the classroom, the community, or a patient care setting. For example, if you are precepting a student in a clinical setting and he's just learning to be reflective, you might prime him to try being continually alert to the thoughts that are passing through his mind, the feelings he is experiencing, and what he imagines his patients are thinking and feeling at various times. If you are tutoring students in a problem-based learning group, questions that you might ask include the following:

- What do I already know that I can bring to bear on this case?
- What are my learning issues?

(Learning issues are unanswered questions that learners want to pursue and topics they want and need to learn more about.)

DURING THE EXPERIENCE

As we've discussed, learners need worthy experiences on which to reflect. In a classroom setting, a learner might do a procedure on a model, engage in role-play, or work with a group of learners on solving a problem. Outside the classroom, in clinical and community settings, almost anything that learners do can provide a springboard for reflection.

If patients will be involved in the learning experience, explain to them what will be happening and get their informed consent, if appropriate.   In many teaching facilities, such as university hospitals, patients are informed that some of their care may be provided by learners who are supervised by seasoned clinicians. Such information can be helpful, but patients are likely to be most comfortable if you or the learner also explain your respective roles, and describe the kinds of educational interactions that will occur. For example, after expressing your confidence in the student's skills, you might explain that the student will do a particular procedure and that you and the student will be talking aloud about what she is doing. You can also let the patient know that you will invite his questions and comments. Or, as another example, if a student will examine and talk with the patient before you join them, the student can explain each of your roles to the patient. Then he can explain that you will be joining them and supervising him.

Invite the learner to talk about what he or she is thinking and doing, if appropriate.   You can help learners practice reflection-in-action and see its benefits by inviting them to think aloud while doing tasks that you are supervising. This can work well in simulations during which learners can do what Arendt (1971) calls "stop-and-think." It can also work well when learners are doing simple, straightforward procedures during which they can easily talk while working. Of course, if a procedure could be harmful if done incorrectly, you can ask the learners to say aloud what they intend to do, then pause so you either support their plan or provide corrective feedback.

If appropriate, help learners consider other approaches.
With some procedures and simulations, after learners tell you what they intend to do next, you can take a few moments to invite them to explain their rationale for what they want to do. In some cases, you might even ask them to suggest other options. Having them reflect this way, even if they have proposed a correct approach, can

help them refine their thinking and establish the mind-set of being routinely reflective. With some procedures, however, there may not be time for such an exchange, so you may need to simply give them immediate feedback. If, for example, you are supervising a learner during a surgical procedure, your corrective feedback may be urgently needed, and providing time for the learner's reflections on possible alternative approaches may not be appropriate.

When you join learners and their patients after they have done a workup and formulated a plan, you can still help them consider options. For example, if a student tells you she thinks that the patient has an allergic rash, but you suspect the findings are a complication of diabetes, you could say, "Given what Ms. Jones reported, I can understand you considering an allergic rash. Can you think of anything else that might present with these symptoms and findings?"

Support the learners' relationships with their patients. When you join a learner who is already talking with a patient, the patient may try to shift the focus away from the learner to you. She might, for example, turn and ask you a question. To keep the focus on the learner, you have several options. One is to turn to the learner when a patient asks you a question, indicating nonverbally that you want the learner to answer. If the patient tries looking at you but cannot make eye contact, she will most likely look where you are looking—at the learner. The learner can then comfortably reply. If your nonverbal cue proves insufficient, you could also ask the student, "What do you think?" At times it's appropriate to respond directly to patients. Usually, it's best though to enable the learner to be the first to respond.

When you feel satisfied that the learner is on the right track, you can let the student and patient know that you endorse the direction in which they are moving and excuse yourself.

AFTER THE EXPERIENCES

Even if you interacted with learners during an activity, you can provide additional help afterwards by reflecting with them on what transpired. A delayed discussion is particularly desirable if the learner was interacting with a simulated or real patient and there were issues that you didn't want to bring up in the patient's presence. It's especially important to invite learners' reflections if you did not interact with them while they were engaged in the activity.

Begin by inviting the learners' reflections.   If you watch learners engage in an activity, you may be tempted to give them feedback immediately afterwards. As we explain in Chapter 2, however, this approach can deny learners the valuable opportunity of practicing reflection without being influenced by your thinking. Most people feel more comfortable pointing out their areas of weakness themselves, rather than hearing about them from others. Also, when we begin by inviting the learners' reflections and critique, we gain access to important diagnostic information about their levels of candor, insight, and professional comfort as well as their capacity to be reflective and to critique their work accurately. All this information is vital for guiding the instructional choices we then make.

Consider inviting learners to write down their reactions or fill out a form.   Simply encouraging learners to talk about their experience can often work well. If you or they would like a record of their immediate reflections, however, or if several learners have participated simultaneously in the same experience, consider asking all of them to write down their initial reflections before inviting discussion. They could write what first comes to their minds or you can guide their responses with written or oral questions or by asking them to complete an assessment form. Without this step in a group situation, those who don't talk first may lose access to their initial thoughts, and a potentially valuable learning opportunity will be diminished or lost.

Invite learners to reflect on one or more of the following:

Their overall impressions.   Beginning with an open-ended approach encourages learners to acknowledge a range of feelings and thoughts, including negative ones that if left unexplored could get in the way of their learning. For example, a student might have gone into a patient interview with the intention of eliciting a history in a more organized way. However, when the student emerges from the interview his first reflection might be, "My patient kept telling me how angry she was that she had been kept waiting. I told her that I was sorry, but it was really hard to talk with her. I was so upset that I forgot about trying to be more organized."

Any new issues or learning goals that emerged. It is not uncommon for unexpected issues to emerge during learning events, as one did for the student in the previous example. This student might decide that in addition to reflecting on how he elicited information from the patient, he also wants to reflect on why he was so thrown by the patient's anger and how he might better deal with such situations in the future.

In problem-based learning as students jointly work on a paper-based patient care situation or other clinical challenge, they identify learning issues—questions for which none of the members of the group have answers. These issues are the basis for further learning.

Fruitful experiences can bring up sources of confusion, intriguing questions, and new areas of interest. Let learners know that being curious is one of the marks of a mature learner.

What they did well. Too often, review sessions focus exclusively on learners' problem areas. Although learners must recognize what areas need their further attention, they also must know what they are doing well. With feedback we can help learners identify their strengths so that they can preserve, nurture, and build on these capabilities. Given the arduous, often discouraging process of becoming a health professional, we have an extra obligation to help learners be aware of—and feel good about—their accomplishments. Learners are likely to function best and gain the most from experiences when they feel comfortable with themselves and the progress they are making. In a review session, if you anticipate that a learner will focus only on her deficits, ignoring what she did well, you might want to ask her to begin her reflections by identifying at least one thing that she did well or feels good about.

What they were thinking. As learners try to solve paper-based cases or work with real or standardized patients, they are likely to engage in numerous mental processes. For example, if they are trying to arrive at a diagnosis, they may consider and pursue several options before arriving at their conclusion. It's possible though, in some situations, for learners (and practitioners) to arrive at a correct conclusion with mistaken information or faulty reasoning.

It's not uncommon for beginners to be so overwhelmed by the experience of caring for a patient or working through a problem that afterwards they are unaware of what they were thinking or the sequence of their thoughts. Even experienced learners and practitioners can be insufficiently unaware of their mental processes.

To become and remain competent, practitioners need to be aware of and be in the habit of reflecting critically upon their thought processes so they can identify errors in their thinking and make needed changes or seek help. You can help learners get into this habit by asking them to reflect aloud about what they were thinking.

Even if we observed learners while they were engaged in the experience they are critiquing, we can't know what they were thinking unless they were thinking aloud. If you are curious about what a learner was thinking, you can say something like, "You were silent after the patient described her pain. Can you recall what you were thinking?"

As we've discussed, a video recording of the event can be a powerful tool for helping learners remember what they were thinking.

Key decision points and options that were available. When helping learners examine their thinking, it's important to ensure that they've considered the options that are available to them and their patients. Abraham Maslow has been credited with saying, "If the only tool you have is a hammer, you will see every problem as a nail" (Ellen Maslow, Personal Communication, 2000). To be competent, practitioners must have a rich array of tools, or options, available for their use. Learners need to acquire many strategies and recognize the conditions under which each is appropriately used.

Frequently during problem solving exercises, interviews, counseling sessions, and other patient-care tasks there are key decision points at which experienced, reflective practitioners recognize that there are two or more options (tools) to choose from. For example, after some brief introductions, a patient encounter might proceed as follows:

Student: How can I help you today?
Patient: I've been having horrible headaches.

One option is to continue being open-ended and inclusive:

Student: I want to hear about your headaches, but first, is there anything else you're hoping we'll deal with today?

Alternatively, the student could be open-ended but somewhat focused by nodding and indicating an interest in hearing more about this topic, for instance by saying, "Please go on." Or she could choose to be more focused and say, "Please tell me about your headaches."

The student could also choose to be very focused and use questions that are likely to elicit short answers, such as, "When did your headaches begin?"

This example illustrates a decision point involving the process of gathering information. Practitioners face many types of decision points, such as choosing what relationship style to use, how much information to provide, or which treatment plan to recommend.

At most decision points some choices are more desirable than others. Sometimes there is just one clearly optimal choice. Patient care, however, can be highly complex and context-specific. Seasoned, reflective practitioners sometimes decide that the current recommendations based on available evidence simply don't apply to the unique circumstances of the patient they are caring for at the moment (Fischer, 1999).

To help those you supervise learn to wrestle with these complexities, consider inviting them to identify a key decision point in the experience they're reflecting on. (Some students might need help doing this.) Then explore the possible pros and cons of whatever they chose to do. Also ask them to reflect on other options that were available and the possible pros and cons of these options, including any research evidence that is available. (We discuss how groups of students can jointly consider options in Chapter 7.)

Any assumptions, values, or biases that might have affected their behavior. In Chapter 1, we discussed how learners' and practitioners' assumptions, values, and biases can affect their care of patients. Particularly if you suspect that the learner is operating on the basis of unrecognized or unexamined assumptions, values or biases, ask questions like, "You said that you didn't think it was necessary to ask your patient any further questions about how she received the bruises on her face. Can you think of any assumptions that might underlie your decision?"

What they were feeling. Providing health care is more than a cognitive task. As we also discussed in Chapter 1, learners' and practitioners' feelings affect how they interact with patients, family members, colleagues, and others and can even block them from being empathic and saying or doing what is needed. A practitioner who is uncomfortable with strong emotions might change the subject or provide false reassurance if a patient with a newly discovered breast lump starts crying and expresses her fear that the lump might be malignant.

From time to time, all of us react to others with strong feelings that are out of proportion to the objective situation. These reactions are often linked to our prior experiences with other people, especially family members or other important people in our lives. A learner who has very strong emotional ties to her grandmother might find it especially difficult to acknowledge and deal with the impending death of an elderly female patient. A member of a health care team might have trouble challenging the treatment plan proposed by his colleague because the colleague reminds him of an uncle who intimidated him as a child. As part of helping learners become insightful professionals, we can help them look for clues to the source of any reaction they have that doesn't seem appropriate to the current situation.

Learners also need to understand that their own feelings can be a clue to what is going on with their patients. For example, it's not unusual to start feeling a little down when working with depressed patients. Self-aware practitioners can use themselves as instruments of diagnosis and therapy (Balint, 1972; Novack et al., 1997).

Many health professions students are far more comfortable talking about their thoughts than their feelings. Before some of them will be willing to talk about their feelings, they may need to understand the rationale for doing so. If a student is not in touch with her feelings and they appear to be negatively affecting the care she is giving, she may need more help than can be provided in an instructional situation. In some programs, mental health professionals are available to help with such situations.

What they thought the patient, or others who were part of the experience, were thinking and feeling. We can help learners become more sensitive to the needs of patients by asking them to speculate about what the patient was thinking and feeling at key times during a clinical encounter. We discuss ways that learners can check out the validity of these perceptions in Chapter 8. Similarly, if the learning experience included the patient's family or others, asking learners to try to step into the shoes of these people and imagine what they might have been thinking or feeling can help increase the learners' appreciation of other perspectives.

What they need to work on. Students and seasoned practitioners as well need to know that learning to provide high-quality care is a never-ending challenge, and that we expect all of them to have deficiencies and learning needs. When learners identify areas that they need to work on, we can congratulate them for being self-aware. However, if some learners come up with an overwhelming list of areas that they feel need attention, you might want to advise them to not try working on everything at once. You might also want to help them determine which areas need immediate attention and which can be deferred. If learners think they don't have anything to work on, you have an even greater challenge. You will probably need to give them appropriate feedback.

Stretch the learner. As learners reflect on their work, we need to help them see things they may not have noticed. For example, say a teacher is aware that during a patient interview the resident that she was precepting continuously looked at the chart instead of at the patient. The teacher might check to see if the resident merely forgot to mention this in his self-critique or whether it was something he was not aware of.

Also, encourage learners to go as far as possible in their thinking, with comments and questions like the following:

- "Good start. Anything else?"
- "That's an important insight. What about . . . ?"

Use questions to engage and sustain learners' interest and to stimulate, expand, and refine their thinking. For example:

- "What factors did you consider in selecting that medication?"
- "If this patient were a teenager instead of middle-aged, what would you suggest doing?"

Try asking just one question at a time. Avoid questions that are leading or that put learners on the spot and seem intended to "catch" them. Avoid guess-what-I'm thinking questions, in which you ask for answers based on assumptions or premises that you haven't revealed. Such questions are not helpful and can defeat whatever trust you've earned.

You can avoid questions that trick or patronize learners by engaging them in a dialogue rather than a question-and-answer exchange. You might ask, "Is there anything more that *you* want to know before coming up with a plan?" If the student replies, no and you think more information is needed, you might say, "I still don't think that I know enough about. . . . What do you think?"

In general, ask rather than tell. After posing a question, pause and give learners sufficient time to respond. (For more on asking questions, see Westberg & Jason, 1993.)

Ensure that learners have the concepts, language, and questions that they need for reflecting on their work.
Regardless of the kind of experience that learners are reflecting on, they need tools that will enable them to think and talk more clearly about what they are doing. For patient examinations, for example, they may need anatomical terms and positional concepts such as lateral and medial. They also need to know technical terms such as the names of instruments they are using. To reflect on and talk about complex human interactions, they need to be familiar with such concepts as open-ended versus closed questions, or empathic as opposed to sympathetic responses.

If you discover that learners need some tools for reflection, devise a way of helping them get these tools. For instance, before having students critique their first interview with a simulated patient, consider reviewing a videotape with them of a practitioner (perhaps you) interacting with a patient. During this review introduce helpful language and concepts, and give learners practice using these words.

Earlier we observed that learners need to have some questions to ask themselves while engaging in learning experiences. The same or other questions can also be useful following such experiences.

Share your reflections and feedback when appropriate.
Whether you watch learners engage in an experience or hear them describe the experience, you are likely to have observations, ideas, suggestions, and assessments regarding that experience that you'd like to share with them. We recommend helping them make these discoveries for themselves, whenever possible. (In this chapter we focus on some ways to do this.)

As we've mentioned, the review process is best when it is a dialogue, not a monologue. Even after you draw learners out, there are likely to be some issues they don't mention but that you'd like to discuss with them. When and how to do this is the focus of the next chapter.

Reflect with learners on their reflections and self-assessments. As when learning any new skill, students and residents need to assess their progress in developing reflection skills. They are also likely to need your feedback. Particularly if they are new to reflection and self-assessment, consider asking learners at the end of a review session to assess how they did. Then give them feedback on their self-assessment. For example, say a student seemed to be overly hard on herself regarding the way she did a procedure, you might start by gently saying something like, "I have a different view of what happened."

As we've suggested before, you can help learners work on their self-assessment skills by having them and you independently complete parallel assessment forms and then compare the student's responses with yours. Discrepancies between your assessments can provide a good starting place for discussions about the learner's self-assessment skills.

Help learners move toward more balanced views of themselves, if appropriate. Learners who are routinely overcritical of themselves and their work may need help in feeling better about themselves. Learners who have an inflated sense of their capabilities may need help becoming more aware of their limitations and learning needs. For the sake of their professional futures, learners at both ends of this continuum need help to become more accurate self-assessors. Of course, with these and other limitations we identify in our learners, we must be careful not to burden ourselves with unrealistic goals. Not all learner characteristics and difficulties are amenable to modification within the limits of the time and circumstances in which we work with them as teachers.

Invite learners to identify lessons they've learned and learning issues they want to pursue. At the end of a review session in which you have fostered the learners' self-reflection and provided your reflections and feedback, consider asking them to state one or two key things that they will take away from the session. Even ask them to write down these learnings. When students and residents summarize and put emphasis on important learnings, they increase the likelihood of remembering them. To further ensure that they will retain new knowledge and skills, assist learners in linking what they've just learned to what they already know and help them to generalize from particular situations. When appropriate, encourage learners to think through their plans for what they will now do differently as a result of what they've learned. Ask them for the specifics of where and when they will put these lessons into practice.

Also ask learners to identify learning issues that have emerged, and ask them how they can pursue these issues. For example a student might say that he is going to pursue an unanswered question by doing an Internet search on MEDLINE. If needed, help learners identify available resources.

Talking about their learning issues and how they will pursue these issues can help students and residents recognize that learning is ongoing and that they need to take responsibility for their learning. This discussion can be crucial to the long-term value of your work with learners, so be careful to preserve enough time before your session needs to be terminated.

Encourage learners to reflect in a journal or in other written form. Journals have been shown to enhance learners' reflection on their work (Kobert, 1995; Lyons, 1999; Pololi, Frankel, Clay & Jobe, 2001; Riley-Doucet & Wilson, 1997). When working with patients, learners can carry small notebooks, note cards, or perhaps even a notebook or palmtop computer on which they keep records of the issues and problems they want to pursue and the capabilities they want to develop. You can also encourage them to keep a journal in which they record more in-depth reflections, including their feelings related to significant events. Some teachers have learners write brief narratives about meaningful patient care events (Lichstein, 1996).

IN CONCLUSION

One of our central tasks as educators is helping our learners to become practitioners who routinely reflect on their care of patients so that they can provide the best possible care. Some steps for doing this are summarized in the following self-checklist. Whenever possible the learner's self-reflection should be part of a dialogue with us and with others who can offer their perspectives. In the next chapter, we focus on the reflections and feedback that teachers can provide as part of that dialogue.

FOSTERING REFLECTION DURING LEARNING

A Self-Checklist

✔

Before the experience do I . . .

- ☐ discuss any preestablished learning goals?
- ☐ encourage learners to set their own goals?
- ☐ invite learners to assess where they are starting from?
- ☐ encourage learners to have questions ready to ask themselves or suggest some to get them started?

During the experience do I . . .

- ☐ if patients will be involved, explain to them what will be happening and, if appropriate, get their informed consent?
- ☐ invite learners to talk about what they are thinking and doing?
- ☐ help learners consider other approaches, if appropriate?
- ☐ support the learners' relationships with their patients?

After a significant experience do I . . .

- ☐ begin by inviting the learners' reflections?
- ☐ invite learners to write down their reactions or fill out a form?
- ☐ invite learners to reflect on one or more of the following
    - ☐ their overall impressions?
    - ☐ any new issues or goals that emerged?
    - ☐ what they did well?
    - ☐ what they were thinking?
    - ☐ key decision points and options that were available?
    - ☐ any assumptions, values, or biases that might have affected their behavior?

❏   what they were feeling?

❏   what they thought the patient or others who were part of the experience were thinking and feeling?

❏   what they need to work on?

❏   issues and questions that they'd like to pursue?

❏ stretch the learner?

❏ ensure that learners have the concepts, language, and questions they need for reflecting on their work?

❏ share my reflections and feedback when appropriate?

❏ reflect with learners on their reflections and self-assessments?

❏ help learners move toward more balanced views of themselves?

❏ invite learners to identify lessons they've learned and learning issues they want to pursue?

❏ encourage learners to reflect in a journal or in other written form?

CHAPTER 6

Providing Feedback Effectively

Some feedback devices—thermostats, for instance—provide "coupled" feedback. Feedback signals automatically cause predictable changes, such as increasing the output of a heating system so the desired temperature is maintained. Most feedback devices, however, like bathroom scales, fuel gauges, and mirrors provide "uncoupled" feedback that doesn't necessarily result in change because the recipient is free to decide if and how to use it (Porter, 1982).

The feedback that teachers give to learners is uncoupled. Learners' responses to instructional feedback are neither automatic nor predictable. Some learners appreciate the feedback and use it. Others temporarily make changes but then slip back into their old habits. Some learners become defensive. Others thank the feedback provider but change their behavior only when being observed by that person.

For learners to make lasting changes (acquire or refine a skill, modify a habit), they need to be receptive to feedback, and they need to understand and value the recommended changes. Making such changes usually involves a dialogue in which the learner and teacher share their reflections about what took place during the experience and their thoughts about the next steps the learner should take.

In the previous chapter we looked at ways to foster the learner's reflections. As learners develop their reflection skills, they often bring up some of the very issues on which we wanted to give them feedback. This can be a happy circumstance, indicating that the learners are becoming more perceptive. In such situations our task becomes giving them positive feedback on their self-assessment.

Not all learners, however, are ready for a dialogue. Some can't or don't want to hear our feedback because they are overwhelmed or feel vulnerable and insecure. How can we present our feedback in ways that will maximize the possibility that our learners will understand it and be open to considering it? How can we reduce the risk that learners will try to please us while we're around but not internalize needed changes? How can we help learners to be comfortable enough to question our feedback openly and constructively if they think it is off target? Following are some steps that can help. They build upon the steps we presented in the two previous chapters, including creating trust and routinely beginning review sessions by inviting the learner's reflection.

Encourage learners to invite your feedback.   If learners are to continue enhancing their skills during and after their formal education, they need to value and be in the habit of inviting the reflections and feedback of others. Consider talking with learners about the importance of getting additional perspectives and seeking feedback information that supplements their own. You might tell them that if they want feedback from you, you'll often ask for their thoughts first, but that you'll be glad to then give them your perspectives.

Link your feedback to the learner's goals.   Learners are likely to be most receptive to your feedback if they solicit it or if you connect it to what you and they agreed were their learning goals. For example, you might say, "Earlier you said that you'd like to focus on using open questions in helping patients tell their story. Would you like to focus on that as we review this next interview?"

On the other hand, instructional goals and priorities should not be treated as if they were immutable. If important issues emerge unexpectedly during a session, try remaining flexible. Consider raising these new issues, but acknowledge that you are suggesting a deviation from your plan: "I know we hadn't planned to focus on dealing with over-talkative patients [or whatever the issue is], but earlier you mentioned that you had trouble with such a patient today. Would you like to talk about that?"

Try providing your feedback in a timely way. For at least two major reasons, feedback is usually most helpful when provided as soon after the event as possible. First, to be of practical value, feedback should be provided while there is still time for the recipient to make and practice needed changes. For example, a student can probably make best use of your feedback about her interaction with a patient if the patient is still available for further interaction.

Second, the longer the delay between the experience and the review session, the more likely it is that the learner will have forgotten some of the events that are important to discuss, such as the steps or strategies that she considered but did not act on during the experience. These passing thoughts and associated feelings that are at risk of being lost can be important clues to the learner's level of functioning, and they can be the basis for some of the core issues around which effective feedback can be offered. The emotional dimensions of patient encounters—the learner's fears, discomforts, or feelings toward the patient—become progressively less accessible with the passage of time. Of course, we will only gain access to these subtle but fundamental aspects of functioning if we convey our own comfort in dealing with these matters and convince the student that we have helpful observations to offer, regardless of the timing of our exchange.

There are some circumstances when it is best to postpone feedback. Learners who have just completed a highly stressful experience or who are seriously behind in their schedule are unlikely to be fully receptive to our observations, however well intentioned or insightful they may be. Also, if the feedback you want to provide to a learner involves personal or sensitive issues and others are present, you may decide that it is best to wait to offer your observations until you can talk privately with the student.

Provide the feedback directly to the learner. Providing negative feedback can be uncomfortable for both parties involved, so it can be tempting to give negative feedback through another person or by simply writing it on an evaluation form. Feedback works best, however, when it provided as part of an open discussion in which we invite the learner's reactions and thoughts, and sensitively adjust what we say and how we say it according to the learner's demeanor and readiness.

Try beginning your feedback with positive observations.
After inviting the learners' self-critique, learners are more likely to
be open to our reflections if we can begin our comments with a positive rather than a negative observation. Doing this can be especially
important if learners are uneasy, defensive, or excessively self-critical
or if you are working with them for the first time. We are not suggesting that you distort the truth or compromise your convictions
just to find something positive to say. Usually it's possible to find
something positive about most learners' efforts, achievement,
self-assessments, or openness. Your positive observation might even
provide a bridge to discussing a problem. For example:

- "It's good you recognized that your participation in the group
  discussion wasn't optimal."
- I'm glad you're eager to do a good job so let's look at ways to
  improve your report."

Some experts on feedback recommend using the "sandwich"
approach: beginning and ending your observations with positive
comments and putting your negative comments in the middle. This
approach can be helpful with some learners, particularly if you and
the student have not yet developed a trusting relationship. However,
if you use this approach repeatedly there is a risk that some learners
will not fully hear your positive statements because they are antici-
pating the negative critique they know is coming. In addition, learners may discount your positive statements if they suspect that you
are only following a formula.

As always, try accommodating to the unique needs and characteristics of each student. If you aren't sure what your learners prefer
and need, ask them.

Provide concrete, descriptive examples.   Negative labels can be
hurtful and don't guide learners toward needed changes. Learners
are much more likely to be willing to change their behavior if,
instead of assigning negative labels, we describe their behavior as
objectively and neutrally as possible and are genuinely open to an
explanation from them. Instead of telling a student that she is
unprofessional, for instance, the teacher can describe whatever
behavior suggests that label: "Last week you were late to work 3
times and never offered an explanation. And you haven't been

returning calls to patients in a timely way. Can you help me understand what's going on?"

The student might have a satisfactory explanation for her behavior, but if not she is given the opportunity to assess and even name her behavior. This can give her some confidence and self-respect. Also, the focus is on behavior that she can modify, not on her character. If the teacher is open to an explanation and presents the feedback in a neutral way, the student is likely to be open to hearing what is said to her.

Another strategy, particularly for learners who have insight into their behavior, is asking them to describe their behavior. Instead of telling a student that he is insensitive, a teacher and student might have the following exchange:

Teacher: Did you notice what Ms. Jones was doing when you told her that she got herpes because she had been "sleeping around"?

Student: I think she was looking at the floor.

Teacher: How do you think she might have been feeling?

Student: [Pause] She was probably uncomfortable. I guess I sounded accusatory, didn't I?

Concrete examples can also enrich positive feedback and can help learners be aware of behaviors that are desirable. Rather than just being told that he is terrific, a student will likely learn more if he is told why he is well regarded. Commenting on a students' performance in a PBL tutorial session a teacher might say, "I appreciate the way you try to make sure that everyone in the group has a chance to speak."

In a study of students' and faculty members' perceptions of feedback on a clinical clerkship, Gil, Heins, and Jones (1984) found that the students valued feedback. However, the students reported that specific points concerning needed improvements were not emphasized enough and were not made early enough during the clerkship to enable them to make improvements. In addition, they perceived their teachers' feedback to be generally inadequate, vague, and nonspecific.

Consider illustrating your feedback with a video recording of the student. A powerful way to give learners objective feedback about their performance is recording their work on videotape and then reviewing the recording with them. This strategy is particularly helpful when reviewing simulated or real patient encounters. Reviewing recordings increases the likelihood learners will believe— even act on—the critique you provide. In addition, as discussed in the previous chapter, they are likely to recognize many issues for themselves before you provide your critique. (For an extended discussion of using video recordings for providing feedback, see Westberg & Jason, 1994b.)

When your feedback is subjective, label it as such. In some patient record-keeping systems, clinicians are expected to provide their subjective observations. This acknowledges that even when we are trying to provide objective descriptions of people and events, we are likely to be selective in what we perceive and in how we interpret events. Subjectivity is equally inescapable in our work with learners.

You can acknowledge the subjectivity of your feedback by using "I" statements. Instead of presenting assertions as though they were unarguably true ("You were repeatedly preoccupied when the patient tried to. . . ."), consider prefacing your remarks with phrases like the following:

- "I thought that you were . . ."
- "In my view . . ."
- "From my perspective . . ."
- "It seems to me that . . ."

By labeling subjective feedback as deriving from your point of view, you imply that your feedback is not necessarily the final word, and you invite learners to consider challenging your judgment—an important step in their professional maturation. Acknowledging the subjectivity of our observations and hypotheses enhances our credibility, increases the likelihood that learners will be trusting and receptive toward our contributions, and provides learners with a model worth emulating.

When possible, link your feedback to your actual observations of learners. In Chapter 4 we discussed the importance of trying to observe learners as they engage in the activities that will be the subject of their reflection. By observing learners in action, either directly or indirectly via video recordings, you are in a position to provide them with a cross-check of their self-critique. You may also become aware of other important issues that merit discussion.

It isn't possible or necessary to observe a student all the time. As you sense that a student is on the road to being *consciously competent,* you can give him progressively more independence. Even advanced students, though, deserve to be directly observed occasionally. Watching them in action can give you ideas about ways to help them refine and sharpen their skills further. Doing so also allows you to see if they have unknowingly backslid.

Check out any hypotheses you generate about the learner's performance. Our observations of learners interacting with patients or others often will leave us with some *hypotheses*—not clear-cut conclusions—about the learners' intentions and capabilities. Let's say you observe a student interrupt a patient who seems eager to talk about the stress he is feeling at work and that this interruption shifts the discussion back to the particulars about the patient's abdominal complaints. On the surface, this student appears to be insensitive, uncomfortable, or unaware of the importance of personal life experiences in the genesis of symptoms. Yet these possibilities are only hypotheses in need of exploration. Before you give this student any feedback based on your observations, you will likely be most helpful if you first determine his view of the interaction you witnessed. You may learn that during a previous interview, which you did not see, the student had a detailed discussion about the patient's stress at work. Now the student feels he needs to return to the patient's presenting complaint. Contrary to initial appearances, this student may be quite sensitive to the issues that you worried might be a problem for him.

Try to avoid sweeping judgments about learners. Labeling learners with general terms such as incompetent, inadequate or insensitive can make them feel they are being attacked and reduces the possibility that they will reveal their concerns or be open to recommendations for change. Besides, such words can mean many different things, so learners are unlikely to fully understand what the speaker means when he or she labels them with these or similar words. Without specific descriptions to explain why they are being judged in this way, learners may decide that the feedback is incorrect or irrelevant. Or they may feel so distressed by such judgments that they can't derive much constructive benefit from anything else that transpires in the session.

Residents in a study by Hewson and Little (1998) reported that they perceived feedback from teachers as unhelpful and unfair when it made them feel slighted, abused, blamed, or rejected. The residents were put off by teachers' personal judgments, such as "You're obsessive-compulsive," "You're narrow-minded," and "Doctors ought to shut up."

Positive labels are rarely hurtful. Used alone though, they're generally not particularly helpful either. Learners are likely to enjoy being told that they are wonderful or smart, but these labels don't provide them with any guidance or direction.

Labeling learners can be tempting. Doing so can appear to simplify our lives. Most people, however, are enormously complex and can't be reduced to labels. In addition, once learners have been labeled, there is a risk that other teachers (and even the learners themselves) will perceive only those aspects of the learners' behavior that are consistent with the label they've been given.

Avoid premature feedback even when learners do well.
When learners handle a difficult situation especially well, we may be tempted to bypass the first step of inviting their reflections and begin by saying how well they did. Yet whenever we offer our feedback immediately, we risk denying students and residents the learning opportunity associated with being the first to critique their own work. And we run the risk of being incorrect. Also, if we begin a review session by telling a student that he did a marvelous job, he may withhold his concerns and negative self-critique fearing such self-disclosures could diminish the good image we've just formed of him.

There are ways we can invite the learner's reflections and still convey sensitivity to the difficulty of the situation that she has just faced. The following statement does not carry any judgment about the student's performance, yet still expresses sensitivity and support: "That was a very challenging situation. I would have had a difficult time dealing with that patient's level of anger."

Such a statement, if it's true, accomplishes several goals. It reveals your humanness and vulnerability, which contributes to your credibility and trustworthiness. It avoids the possibility of stifling the learner's self-critique. And, if the student experienced some discomfort with the patient's behavior and felt some embarrassment about her discomfort, your revelation may increase her willingness to acknowledge her concerns.

This caution about avoiding premature feedback applies particularly to learners you are just getting to know. If you know a learner well and feel that she trusts you and is not likely to be stifled by your opinions and feedback, postponing your views is less critical.

Avoid overloading learners with feedback. When giving feedback to learners, we may be tempted to convey all the observations that have occurred to us. We can usually be most helpful, however, by squelching that inclination. Most learners, especially those in the early stages of their development, can deal with only one topic at a time. Many can deal with only a few issues in the course of an entire supervisory session. Feedback from a teacher—especially feedback that has negative components—can feel fairly heavy. Time and space are needed for integrating such critique. Also, items that seem simple and straightforward to experienced clinicians can appear quite complicated to neophytes who need time to fully understand and integrate information about changes they will need to make.

Consider prioritizing the issues, focusing on only a few high-priority concerns and putting the other issues aside at least temporarily. If you make notes of what you have already discussed and what you'd like to discuss in the future, you can continue your critique in subsequent meetings. As with patients, continuity of care with learners leads to a better understanding of their backgrounds, characteristics, and needs. With patients or learners who you see repeatedly, you don't have to do or say everything in any one encounter.

Be aware that learners have varying levels of receptivity to feedback. Learners' receptivity to feedback is a critical variable in the mix of factors that determine the success of supervisory sessions. Any individual's level of receptivity can be the product of recent and past events. If a student has just emerged from a traumatic experience with a patient or has recently received a large dose of negative feedback from another teacher, he will probably not be open to additional feedback at this time. In order to decide the timing and amount of the feedback you will offer, take into account the learner's recent experiences and current emotional and intellectual state. In some situations, you may want to consider saying something like, "I have some feedback for you. Would this be a good time?" If you have earned some measure of trust from this learner, you are likely to get a straight answer.

Convey your support when providing feedback. If we convey support for learners, even while expressing our concerns about problems that have emerged in their work, our contributions are likely to be heard, valued, and assimilated. If learners perceive us as indifferent or disdainful, our feedback will be less helpful than it could have been. What we say and how we say it are important. Our body language, tone, and pacing can be even more important than the specific words we use (Tannen, 1990).

Check for understanding and invite the learners' reactions to your feedback. Teachers risk not being heard or understood when they present their observations and comments without confirming that their learners have understood them. They may even have an unintended impact.

After giving feedback to learners, we can facilitate a dialogue with comments like:

- "That's what I observed. What's your perception of what happened?"
- "Please give me your candid reaction to my feedback."

The learners' perceptions of what happened may be different from ours, and they might help us see things that we missed. The learners' reactions can also provide us with clues to their readiness for and receptivity to our feedback. Their reactions can also help us determine whether they heard and understood what we said.

Help learners turn negative feedback into constructive challenges. Giving corrective feedback to learners in ways that help them feel constructively challenged—not demeaned or assaulted—can be difficult. You can begin by reminding them that we expect all learners to have skills they need to work on. Why else would they be in an educational program? You can also help them reframe negative feedback into learning goals and think through some specific strategies for reaching those goals.

Whenever possible, link your feedback to the goals to which learners have said they are committed. For instance: "We talked about how you've been interrupting patients and how you want to learn to give them space so they can tell you what's bothering them. Can you think of some ways to learn to do that?"

Provide follow-up to your feedback whenever appropriate. After giving feedback, particularly negative feedback, your task may not be done. In many situations we need to help students develop a plan for dealing with whatever problems or deficiencies we have identified together. If follow-up is appropriate and possible, you may also need to arrange a way to monitor your learners' progress. Careful planning and follow-up are particularly important if your feedback has a strong emotional impact on the learner. If, for example, you convey the news that the student will probably not pass the course, or if your feedback led to the recognition that your learner is depressed or has another serious personal problem, you need to provide or arrange for careful follow-up. Even in less dramatic or serious situations, follow-up is often indicated.

Little if any meaningful change in human behavior occurs as the result of a single, brief intervention. Providing follow-up can reinforce and ensure the lasting, positive outcomes your feedback is meant to achieve. It can also help avoid any undesirable consequences of feedback.

IN CONCLUSION

Timely, constructive feedback is essential to learning. Yet too often learners don't get the feedback they need, and some of the feedback they get is delivered too late and in hurtful ways. We suggest some steps for providing feedback effectively. We stress the importance of first inviting the learner's reflections and engaging in a dialogue rather than a monologue. If learners are to provide high-quality care throughout their careers, they need to value and invite feedback from trusted colleagues. If you help them value feedback and provide them with useful feedback, they may well begin reaching out to you and others for feedback throughout their formal education.

PROVIDING FEEDBACK EFFECTIVELY

A Self-Checklist

❑ ✔

Do I . . .

❑   begin by inviting the learners' reflections?

❑   encourage learners to invite my feedback?

❑   link my feedback to each learner's goals?

❑   try to provide my feedback in a timely way?

❑   provide the feedback directly to the learner?

❑   try beginning my feedback with positive observations?

❑   provide concrete, descriptive examples?

❑   consider illustrating my feedback with a video recording of the student?

❑   label my feedback as subjective when it is?

❑   link my feedback to my actual observations of learners when possible?

❑   check out any hypotheses I generate about the learner's performance?

❑   try to avoid sweeping judgments about learners?

❑   avoid premature feedback even when learners do well?

❑   avoid overloading learners with feedback?

❑   recognize that learners have varying levels of receptivity to feedback?

❑   convey my support when providing feedback?

❑   check for understanding and invite the learners' reaction to my feedback?

❑   help learners turn negative feedback into constructive challenges?

❑   provide follow-up to my feedback whenever appropriate?

CHAPTER **7**

Helping Learners Reflect
With and Give Feedback
to Each Other

C ollective reflection and feedback can take many forms. Here
we focus on students, residents, or practitioners meeting in
small groups to reflect on *individual* and *shared* experiences.
In some programs small groups of students who have different clinical assignments in the community meet at regular intervals to
reflect aloud on questions, ideas, observations, and feelings that
have been stimulated by their individual experiences with patients
and families. The students also invite the perspectives and feedback
of others in the group. Another example of collective reflection on
individual experiences is nursing students who, following their
patient-care tasks in a hospital or health care center, attend confer-
ences where similar exchanges occur. Still another example is Balint
groups, which are made up of physicians (residents or community
physicians) who meet regularly to reflect on their relationships with
patients, especially those they've found difficult to work with (Botelho,
McDaniel, & Jones, 1990).

Groups or teams of learners or practitioners also meet to reflect
collectively and give feedback to one another regarding their *shared*
experiences. Some problem-based learning tutorial groups routinely
take a few minutes at the end of each session to review their
progress in learning from their current case and to reflect on how
they are working together. Other examples are students working as

a team on community projects who reflect on the outcomes and processes of their joint work and learners on health teams who collectively reflect on their shared care of a patient.

Medical teaching rounds can include collective reflection and constructive feedback. Often though, competitive environments make it difficult for students and residents to talk openly about their anxieties and other feelings. Learners may even be reluctant to ask questions or propose options for fear they will reveal their ignorance, which will be used against them. Too often feedback is primarily negative and not provided in helpful ways.

When learners reflect together about their individual patient-care experiences, they expand the number of patients to whom they are exposed and from whom they can learn. There are also other potential benefits of collectively reflecting on individual and shared experiences:

- Learners can be stretched and helped by the feedback and perspectives of others.
- When some group members have recently developed the skill that their peer is trying to learn, they are likely to still be *consciously competent* and thus in a position to be especially helpful.
- If learners are to become and remain safe practitioners, they need to learn to share their doubts and uncertainties with trusted colleagues and to seek the perspectives and advice of others.
- Hearing their peers express their self-doubts and uncertainties can be helpful to learners who worry that they are the only ones who have these concerns.

Another benefit of collectively reflecting on experiences is that doing so can help prepare students and residents for working collegially as members of formal and informal health care teams. Members of effectively functioning health teams need to be good at critiquing their own work, giving feedback to colleagues, respecting different perspectives, and negotiating differences. Learners who meet regularly to review individual or common experiences have opportunities to work on these skills.

The basic principles involved in fostering reflection and providing feedback constructively apply in all contexts, including peer learning. Yet peer learning presents some special considerations. Learners' behaviors with each other often mirror their institution's educational culture. Promoting peer learning is likely to be far easier in programs where reflection is valued and learners are treated as emerging professionals than in programs where reflection is devalued and learners are treated as dependent or incompetent. It is also easier to engage learners in constructive collective reflection and feedback in institutions that promote collaboration than in institutions that intentionally or unknowingly foster competition through their evaluation system and interaction patterns.

Following are some suggestions for ways to help learners reflect together and provide feedback to each other. They are built on suggestions provided in Chapters 4 though 6. Some of the steps, such as establishing ground rules, can help reduce or prevent such problems as learners providing feedback in hurtful ways.

Help learners see the value of taking time for collectively reflecting on experiences. Particularly in nonreflective environments, some learners may think that sitting around reflecting on past experiences is a waste of time. Try to determine the extent to which your learners value reflection, or whether they even know what a reflective practitioner is. Consider asking them how they feel about the particular reflection sessions that you intend to conduct. If you haven't yet established an atmosphere of full, trusting openness in your group, you may have to interpret their replies, realizing that they might not feel ready to be fully honest with you.

If they don't know what a reflective practitioner is, spend some time discussing this notion. If you sense that they are skeptical about the value of reflection, invite them to talk about why they feel this way. Also, consider asking them to identify some possible arguments for taking time to reflect on their work. (See Chapter 1 for some ideas.)

Helping skeptical learners gain some understanding of the rationale for reflection can be a valuable start. Before they become committed to the idea, however, they will likely need repeated opportunities to experience its value for them and their learning.

Discuss the format that you will use in the session. The format will depend on whether the group is reflecting on individual or common experiences, whether video recordings are being used, the amount of time you have available, and other factors. We recommend that learners reflect on their own work before inviting feedback from their peers and from you. If you will be following this sequence, during your first session consider asking the learners why they think this sequence can be helpful both for them and you. One factor to discuss is that most people are more comfortable identifying their problem areas themselves rather than having someone else do so.

Help the learners create a safe environment for reflection and feedback. Learners are not likely to be open about their needs and perceived deficiencies if they are worried that they will be put down or that this information will be used against them in other ways. Consider talking with them about how most of us are initially uneasy about being candid with others and that it usually takes time to develop trust. If you ask them what the group can do to make the experience of being self-reflective as comfortable as possible, they might say that they would feel more free to talk about problems if what they say is kept confidential.

Consider talking about how most of us are uncomfortable giving and receiving feedback, particularly when it is negative. In some cultures people are also quite uncomfortable giving positive feedback. To guide your work together, ask learners under what conditions your feedback and that of their peers will be most helpful to them. They might say that they are most likely to be open to feedback if it is specific, descriptive, and provided in a supportive way. Consider asking them to write their suggestions on the chalkboard or on a flipchart.

Establish ground rules for your work together. To help ensure that learners will feel as comfortable as possible and to minimize the risk that peers' feedback might be distracting or harmful, ask learners to establish ground rules at the beginning of the first session. You could begin with their suggestions for making the environment as safe as possible. The ground rules that some groups use include the following ideas:

- Begin by asking the person whose work is being discussed to give his reflections.
- Don't talk *about* anyone who isn't present or about a person as if she weren't present (in other words, give feedback directly *to* a person).
- Offer positive observations before negative ones.
- Before giving feedback to someone else, think through what it would be like to the recipient of that feedback.

- Illustrate your points with specific examples based on your observations.
- Withhold your negative observations unless you can offer recommendations for improving the behavior in question.

If a learner is reflecting aloud on his or her experience, ask that person to identify any specific help that he or she would like from the group. Consider talking with the learners about why it might be important for health professionals to be willing and able to ask for feedback and advice from trusted colleagues. Discuss how they can practice doing that with each other. For example, a student in a problem-based tutorial group might say, "I've been trying to listen without interrupting other people, and I've been trying to be clearer when I present ideas and information. What's your impression of how I'm doing?"

If the group is reflecting on a joint experience, consider creating an agenda. Being clear about the issues that need to be addressed can enable a group to make the best use of its time. Prior to the reflection session, you might want to create a list of questions for the group to discuss, or you might want them to come up with their own agenda. For example, after doing a problem-solving exercise together, members can create a list of issues to be discussed and then prioritize the list so they deal first with the most important and pressing issues.

Help students and residents learn to foster each other's self-reflections. Consider talking with the learners about how people tend to have more ownership of their learning when they make their own discoveries. Model some ways of fostering self-reflection, perhaps focusing on the kinds of issues identified in Chapter 5. Give learners some tools for helping their peers be reflective, including questions like the following:

- What were you hoping to accomplish?
- What were you thinking?
- What was it like to be in that situation?
- Have you thought of any other ways that you could handle that kind of situation?

Model ways to foster reflection and provide feedback constructively.   Learners are likely to learn as much or more from the *way* we give feedback as from *what* we say about feedback.

Help learners provide each other with balanced critique. Sometimes during peer review learners focus exclusively on what their colleagues did well, perhaps hoping their colleagues will give them a favorable critique in return. Although this restraint may initially reduce the learners' anxiety, avoiding negative critiques can shortchange the learners whose work is being reviewed, denying them the opportunity to get some potentially important feedback. If this happens, consider modeling constructive, supportive ways of introducing and discussing learners' problem areas.

By contrast, in competitive environments some learners might begin their feedback by focusing on what their colleague did *not* do well and fail to point out what went well. This can create a sense of discomfort that can interfere with establishing a trust-based environment. If you anticipate that learners will focus on the negative, consider asking them to first focus on what went well.

Intervene if peer critique is not constructive.   If a student provides potentially hurtful feedback, intervene quickly or let other members of the group intervene if they are inclined and able to do so. Sometimes it's helpful to invoke the group's ground rules by saying, "Remember one of the ground rules that we agreed to is describing rather than giving negative labels to our perceptions of what happened."

The early stages in establishing a system for regular peer review must go smoothly and be perceived by all participants as genuinely helpful, or learners may withdraw—partly or fully—and a potentially valuable set of learning experiences will have been lost.

Encourage learners to seek alternative perspectives and strategies.   One of the advantages of collective reflection is that students and residents can learn from each other. After a learner has reflected on what she did in the situation being reviewed and she has considered other ways that she might have dealt with the situation, encourage her to ask other members of the group if they have other perspectives or alternative strategies to recommend. This gives the learner practice in turning for help to colleagues, a desirable habit for life-long learning. And because she has made the request she is less likely to feel demeaned by others who foist their ideas on her, perhaps in an attempt to elevate themselves at her expense. To increase the likelihood that learners will try other approaches, consider inviting learners to role-play with each other—in effect, rehearse—what they could say or do in future patient-care situations.

Help learners extract general principles and strategies.   Irby (1986) contends that the weakest link in experiential clinical learning is "generalizing from the particular experiences to a general principle applicable in other circumstances" (p. 36). Postexperience discussion and reflection, he says, is critical to the learning process because it enables learners to infer general principles from their experiences. To help learners extract general principles and strategies from their own experiences and the experiences of their peers, you can ask questions such as:

- "How would you describe the strategy that John used?"
- "Have any of you used that kind of strategy in other situations? If so, what did you do and how did it work?"
- "Can you think of any future situations where that strategy could be useful?"

Invite learners to reflect on the process of the session in which you have just engaged and how you might do better in the next session.   Ongoing groups are dynamic organisms that grow and change. In the first stage of group development, members typically aren't sure what they are supposed to do. In the second stage they struggle with the group's tasks and with how they will work together. If conflicts are resolved, groups move to the third stage, which is characterized by trust and harmony, and then to the fourth stage, which is characterized by productivity. (See Westberg & Jason, 1996 for various descriptions of the stages of group development.)

To ensure that problems don't fester and that your group evolves to the fourth stage in which learners can get the most out of each session, invite members to think through how all of you worked together, including what went well and what didn't. Here are some questions you might consider asking:

- "How did the format work?"
- "To what extent were you comfortable reflecting out loud about your work and receiving feedback?"
- "If you were not comfortable, what got in the way?"
- "Were you clear about your roles and tasks? If not, what were the sources of confusion?"
- "Did you feel that you were able to participate fully? If not, what got in the way?"

After the learners have shared their reflections, offer yours, including observations of any important events or issues that appear to have escaped their attention. Next, think through together what you want to retain and what changes you want to try during the next session.

Invite learners to summarize what they've learned and the learning issues they want to pursue. As we've discussed, doing these kinds of summaries can help learners retain the lessons they've learned and take responsibility for their ongoing learning. Also, when students or residents make statements in the presence of peers about what they've learned, other members of the group can be reminded of what *they* have learned. Publicly stating how they intend to pursue their learning goals can also enhance the learners' sense of commitment to these goals and improve the chances that they will follow through on their plans.

If the focus of the session was on an individual's experience, that person should probably be the first to summarize his or her questions, learnings, and next steps. Then since peers can learn from each other's experiences, all of the group members should be invited to share what they're taking away from the session. If the focus of the session was on a shared experience, the group members can still talk about their individual questions, learnings, and follow-up steps, but it will probably be important for group members to also identify shared learning issues and to decide who will pursue each issue. For example, in problem-based learning, members of the group divide the learning tasks. Then at their next session, they teach each other what they have learned.

Invite students and residents to reflect on what they already knew and what they learned from each other. As we discussed in Chapter 1, learners build knowledge by linking new understandings to what they already know. Acknowledging what they already knew can be particularly helpful to beginning students in the health professions who sometimes feel that they don't know anything. Hearing about their peers' life experiences can also help members get to know one another better, which can enhance trust and improve their prospects for productive collaboration.

When group members summarize what they've learned, particularly in collaborative environments, they often acknowledge what they've learned from each other. If you have learned something from group members, consider telling them so. These steps can build collegiality and help to underscore the benefits of working and learning with others.

Make arrangements for the next session.   Be sure that everyone is clear about when and where the next session will be held, what preparations members are expected to make for the next session, and what their roles and responsibilities will be during that session. As you think through the learners' roles and responsibilities, be aware that being an effective group facilitator is analogous in many ways to being an effective parent. Our goal is for learners to become increasingly more able to function on their own. Initially we need to provide direction and model what they need to learn. If we do our job well, learners assume progressively more responsibility for their learning, and our role shifts toward being a coach. Eventually we can fade into the background and serve as consultants. To achieve this transition we need to define our success in terms of what learners become able to do for themselves rather than what we do to and for them. (For a detailed discussion of facilitating small groups, see Westberg & Jason, 1996.)

IN CONCLUSION

Collective reflection and feedback has many benefits, including providing learners with different perspectives and preparing them to function as collegial members of health teams. By giving them practice doing self-assessments in the presence of their peers, giving feedback to others, and negotiating differences, we prepare them for collaborative practice. Engaging learners in collective reflection is particularly difficult in institutions where reflection is devalued, students are treated in harsh, demeaning ways, and competition is engendered. Yet even in these environments teachers can create well-functioning groups in which students and residents contribute to one another's learning.

HELPING LEARNERS REFLECT WITH AND GIVE FEEDBACK TO EACH OTHER

A Self-Checklist

❑ ✔

Do I . . .

❑ help learners see the value of taking time for collectively reflecting on experiences?

❑ discuss the format that we will use in the session?

❑ help the learners create a safe environment for reflection and feedback?

❑ help the learners establish ground rules for our work together?

❑ if a learner is reflecting aloud on his or her experience, ask that person to identify any specific help that he or she would like from the group?

❑ if the group is reflecting on a joint experience, consider creating an agenda?

❑ help students and residents learn to foster each other's self-reflections?

❑ model ways to foster reflection and provide feedback constructively?

❑ help learners provide each other with balanced critique?

❑ intervene if any critique is not constructive?

❑ encourage learners to seek alternative perspectives and strategies?

❑ help learners extract general principles and strategies?

❑ invite learners to reflect on the process of the session in which they have just engaged and how the next session can be improved?

❑ invite learners to summarize what they've learned and the learning issues they want to pursue?

❑ invite students and residents to reflect on what they already knew and what they learned from each other?

❑ make arrangements for the next session?

CHAPTER 8

Helping Learners Elicit Feedback From Patients

Patients can and should be among the most important sources of feedback for learners during their formal education and throughout their careers. Since a primary goal of the health professions is helping people, it is crucial to find out whether those being served do feel helped. If patients don't feel that a practitioner or the system is helpful, their concerns deserve to be heard and responded to appropriately.

Increasingly educators are recognizing that the outcomes of health care are most likely to be positive if patients are active participants and partners in their care. Successful partnerships require conversations about what's working and what's not, and what can be done to make the process more successful.

Some practitioners and health care organizations regularly elicit patients' feedback. Typically they do this by giving questionnaires to patients after a hospital visit or a primary care encounter. Or they mail questionnaires to them later.

Some schools and residency programs invite real and standardized patients to help in the educational program (e.g., Kahn, Cohen, & Jason, 1979; O'Connor, Albert, & Thomas, 1999; Stillman, Regan, Philbin, & Haley, 1990). Some community-oriented programs involve community leaders in the education of health professions students (e.g., McGrew & Kaufman, 1999). Most programs, however, don't begin to take full advantage of this rich resource.

After interacting with learners or practitioners, patients are uniquely equipped to provide observations about such matters as the extent to which they felt that the student, resident, or practitioner:

- treated them with dignity and respect
- gave them opportunities to present their concerns
- listened carefully to their concerns
- presented information in language that they could understand
- provided advice that was helpful
- suggested a treatment plan that they can reasonably carry out
- invited and responded to their questions

Patients' reflections are especially valuable because they alone know whether the learner with whom they interacted is someone they can confide in, someone they trust, someone who seems to genuinely care about them. Also they are the only ones who are able to say how it felt when the learner examined them. And only they know whether they are likely to carry out the treatment plan. If several patients give consistent negative feedback—perhaps that a learner doesn't listen carefully to their concerns or doesn't treat them with dignity and respect—that feedback deserves to be explored further.

Students may take patients' feedback more seriously than feedback from teachers, particularly if it pertains to issues that patients are in a good position to evaluate. A learner may resist his teacher's observation that he often uses language that patients can't understand, but he might take quite seriously a patient's observation that she couldn't understand some of the words he used. We've repeatedly found that most learners work hard at making changes that are prompted by what they hear from patients. Studies indicate that a significant number of residents and practitioners make changes based on feedback from patients (Cope, Linn, Leake, & Barrett, 1986; Hearnshaw, Baker, Cooper, & Soper, 1996).

DETERMINING WHEN AND HOW TO ELICIT FEEDBACK FROM PATIENTS

There are several strategies you can use for eliciting feedback from patients.

Ask patients to complete feedback forms. Creating forms that patients can use in assessing the learners' interactions with them can be time-consuming, as can devising ways to get the forms to and from patients. This feedback can be so valuable, however, that we think that the effort is worthwhile. Once the form is created and the mechanisms for getting the data are in place, you can collect the data on many learners over time relatively automatically. If learners find the feedback valuable, they may adapt the form for use later in their own practices.

The forms should be simple and easy to complete, allowing patients to provide information such as the extent to which the learner who cared for them was respectful, listened carefully to what they said, and invited their questions. You can ask learners and patients to help with creating the form. Before the form is used, it should be tested by a variety of patients who are representative of the population being served.

You will need to determine whether the form should be filled out anonymously and whether it will be feasible and useful to collect some demographic information. For instance, if you want to determine if learners are perceived differently by—or behave differently with—various groups of patients, you might want patients to indicate their age range, gender, or other relevant characteristics on the feedback form.

When deciding how to distribute the forms, consider asking the learners or a staff member to give the form to every patient at the end of each visit. Or consider mailing the form to patients along with a stamped, addressed envelope. Figure out a way to assemble the data so that you and the learners can review the patient feedback in a timely and constructive way.

Ask learners to complete parallel assessment forms. Asking learners to complete forms that are parallel to the ones being filled out by patients can enable you and the learners to see the extent to which their self-perceptions match the feedback of patients. If there is a discrepancy between the way that a significant number of patients perceive a learner and the way that learner perceives herself, you may well have an important issue for you and the learner to discuss.

Ask learners to routinely elicit feedback informally. In addition to or instead of written feedback from patients, learners can informally invite direct feedback from patients. During a patient visit in a primary care setting, learners can protect a couple of minutes at the end of each session for asking and responding to patient questions like these:

- "Did you have any concerns that you didn't get to tell me about during our session?"
- "Was there anything I told you that you weren't clear about?"
- "Were there any other questions you wanted to ask me?"

Learners can also elicit feedback during and at the end of a patient's hospital or nursing home stay.

Here are some steps to consider if you ask learners to elicit feedback from patients:

- Ensure that learners understand why it's important to get feedback from patients.
- Model this behavior in the learners' presence.
- Discuss some of the kinds of feedback that patients are uniquely able to give to learners and practitioners.
- Help learners think through some of the specific information they would like to get from patients.
- Have learners formulate questions they'd like to ask and even have them rehearse asking these questions.
- Accompany learners when they first try to elicit feedback from patients so that you and they can later reflect on how this strategy worked and what the learner might want to do differently next time.
- Routinely ask learners if they are eliciting feedback from patients and, if so, what they are learning from their patients.

Consider using standardized patients.   Standardized patients are people who have been trained to present with certain symptoms, historical information, and pertinent issues in their lives. They may withhold some of this information if the learner fails to ask certain questions or if the learner does not communicate effectively. Some standardized patients are also trained to provide constructive feedback.

The role-playing between the learner and the patient can take place in a classroom or a clinical setting. The learner is given a task, say to interview or examine the patient or to provide the patient with information about his condition or proposed treatment. We recommend that the learners be themselves rather than assume a role. Both the learner and the standardized patient are given a context. For example, the patient is coming for the first time to a health center complaining of a headache. Often the role-playing is limited to 5 or 10 minutes, and sometimes it is videotaped.

After the role-play, the learner reviews the experience with the standardized patient or a preceptor or both. Other learners might also be present, and they may join in the review. The review can result in the learner practicing the interaction again, this time trying out one or more lessons that he learned from the first experience.

Standardized patients have been used for teaching in schools in the health professions for decades (Jason et al., 1971; Kahn et al., 1979; O'Connor, Albert, & Thomas, 1999). A growing number of schools are training standardized patients to be available for use in a variety of courses. (For information on how to select and train standardized patients, see Westberg and Jason, 1994b.)

Some of the advantages of having learners use standardized patients when practicing new skills are not having to intrude on real patients and being able to "program" the patients so that they have the specific problems and personal characteristics needed for the learners' practice. Standardized patients who have been trained to provide feedback can give learners useful information in a supportive way. Also, they aren't constrained by the fears held by some real patients that their health care might be jeopardized if they provide negative (honest) feedback. Further, learners can ask standardized patients questions that they wouldn't feel comfortable asking a real patient with whom they have an ongoing relationship. For example, learners may be uneasy asking their real patients if something they did made it difficult for the patient to discuss sensitive issues.

You may want to take some of the following steps if you use standardized patients:

- Be sure the standardized patients understand what kind of information will be most helpful to learners.
- Create a checklist or assessment form that can guide the standardized patient in providing feedback.
- Have the standardized patients rehearse providing feedback before they work with learners.
- Determine the learners' experience and comfort in role-playing with standardized patients and try to address any potential problems.
- After the role-play, ask the learners to share their reflections about the experience before they invite the patient's feedback.

- After the learner and patient have reflected on their interaction, invite the learner to do the role-play again, using the lessons just learned.
- Ask learners to reflect on their experiences of redoing the role-play.

As learners become more aware of the skills they need to develop and the ways that standardized patients can help them do that, they can participate more in preparing the standardized patient and guiding the review. For example, if a resident wants to learn how to deal more effectively with an angry patient, she can request that the patient present as an angry person. During the review of the role-play, she can ask the patient how he felt when she tried different strategies, and she can ask the patient to suggest other strategies that might work in the future.

Invite learners to role-play being a patient. In a classroom setting, consider asking a learner to role-play with another learner who plays the part of a patient. The "patient" can be given a brief script with a few symptoms and a little historical information. As with standardized patients, provide a context. The role-play may be limited to 5 minutes. Then both learners can reflect aloud on the experience from their perspectives.

Most of the benefits that can be derived from role-playing with standardized patients also apply to role-playing with peers. Unlike using standardized patients, peer role-playing doesn't require finding or training a standardized patient, and the role-playing can be done fairly spontaneously. (You can develop a simple scenario on the spot in the midst of a class discussion or other instructional activity.)

A major benefit of peer role-playing is that learners can gain insights from putting themselves in the patient's role. In a role-play in which the "practitioner" is condescending, the learner, who is programmed to be a patient with a sensitive, personal issue might realize how difficult it is to disclose such information to a practitioner who he fears might be dismissive or judgmental. Such experiences can lead to greater empathy for the patient's situation. One disadvantage of peer role-playing is that learners sometimes find it difficult initially to imagine a peer who they know well, as someone else.

As usual, begin by being diagnostic. Determine the learners' experiences and comfort with role-playing with peers and try to address any problems that they've experienced. If you want to focus on the experience of being a patient, consider asking the learner who was the patient to share his or her feelings first. Invite learners to draw on their own experiences as a patient in order to become more empathic with the patient's position. As when role-playing with standardized patients, consider asking the learners to role-play again using lessons they extracted from the initial experience. Encourage them to take the kinds of risks that aren't possible when working with real patients. Then ask the learners to reflect on the second role-play, including how it felt and what worked and what didn't.

Make video recordings of the interaction between the learner and a standardized patient, and invite the patient to review the tape with the learner. Earlier we presented some reasons for using videotape recordings of learners and patients during review sessions at which patients are not present. Some of the same advantages exist when standardized or real patients are present for a videotape review session. Since there is a recording, no one needs to guess what happened during the interaction. The recordings can prompt learners and standardized patients to remember thoughts, feelings, and events that they otherwise might forget partially or completely. And video recordings can help learners, patients, and observers see things that they didn't see the first time around.

Many schools and programs now have their own video equipment, at the very least a monitor you can use with your own or a borrowed camcorder. Set the camera on a tripod and frame the picture so you get the shot you want. (For detailed information on making and using videotapes, see Westberg and Jason, 1994b.)

Before the review session, talk with the learner about this unique opportunity to find out what's going on inside patients during interactions with them. Find out if there's anything in particular that the learner would like to know.

Be sure that the learner and patient are clear about the purposes for reviewing the videotape and about how you and they are going to proceed. Consider asking the patient and the learner to share some of their overall reactions before viewing the tape. This initial step can help you and them be aware of important issues, making it possible for everyone to prioritize the issues and make the best use of your time together.

Consider having the learner operate the remote control but suggest that you or the patient can signal if you want the learner to stop the playback so that you can ask a question or make a comment. These are some of the things you and the learner might want to ask patients to comment on:

- any discomfort or difficulties they had during the encounter
- any thoughts and feelings they experienced but didn't fully express during the original exchange
- examples of approaches used by the learner that they found particularly helpful, distracting, or bothersome
- examples of steps the learner took that made it easier or more difficult for them to say what they had wanted to say

Unless the patient has been trained to give feedback, you may have to take the lead in eliciting feedback, at least initially. As much as possible, though, encourage learners to take responsibility for the session, stopping the tape and inviting the patient's reflections and feedback.

Make video recordings with real patients and invite them to review the tape with the learner. Our focus here is on learners who are in the early stages of their clinical education and patients who are not under the learners' ongoing care. Senior students and residents can review video recordings with patients who are in their care, but doing an in-depth review in a way that doesn't interfere with the learner-patient health care relationship can be tricky and is beyond the scope of what we are addressing here.

If your student will be working with one of your patients, you will probably want to select a patient who you think will be comfortable with the process and able to give students helpful feedback. Some preceptors have sensitive, articulate patients who regularly do this kind of review with students.

If you videotape the interaction in a clinical setting, you may need to find a room where you can have videotape playback equipment and review the tape in privacy without disrupting the clinical schedule. You will also need to obtain the patients' informed consent. In addition, patients need to be informed about what's involved in reviewing the videotape with the learners. A global sense of the purposes of the sessions, an overview of what will happen during the session and what their role will be usually provides them with enough information to decide whether they want to participate.

Many patients feel vulnerable in medical settings, so be sure to discuss any concerns they have about providing feedback. Our experiences and those of others confirm that most patients are willing to provide feedback. In fact, many of them are pleased to be asked. Initially though a few are uneasy about the process, fearing that if they give negative feedback, their future care might be negatively affected. They need to know that regardless of what they say they will be well treated.

Before reviewing the tape, create a friendly, supportive, and respectful climate, for example, by thanking the patient, stating the purposes of the review, and reiterating what they have to offer to the learner's education. The patient is likely to feel even more relaxed if the learner also thanks the patient and makes it clear that she is genuinely eager to hear the patient's feedback.

As with the videotape review with a standardized patient, consider giving the remote control to the learner but tell the patient to signal the learner if she wants him to stop the tape to make a comment or ask a question. Explain that you will do the same.

If you want to get the patient's most candid thoughts, ask for her overall reactions before beginning the review of the tape. You or the learner could say something like this:

- "Before we look at the tape, do you have any general reactions that you'd like to share?"
- "What was that experience like for you?"

Before starting the replay, consider saying something like the following to the patient:

- "As we watch the videotape, signal [learner's name] if you are reminded of any thoughts or feelings you were having that you didn't mention at the time. Also, stop the tape if something that [learner's name] was doing was particularly helpful or bothersome."

If neither the learner nor the patient stops the tape, consider doing so yourself at key points. For example, if the patient begins to look tense in the recording, you could ask the learner to stop the tape and then ask the patient, "Do you remember what you were thinking or feeling at that moment?"

To be sure that patients don't feel under pressure to reveal something that they want to keep private, tell them at the beginning of the session that they should say only what they are comfortable revealing and that you will respect their wishes and not hold it against them if they would rather not talk about something. Later in the session if you suspect that the patient feels under pressure, reiterate this ground rule.

Another way to review the tape is by focusing on one or more issues that the learner has chosen. For example, before starting the tape a student might say, "I'm trying to learn to explain things clearly. Please ask me to stop the tape whenever I'm using language that isn't clear."

Throughout the review session, make sure that the feedback is constructive. Occasionally you will need to protect a learner from nonconstructive feedback. Most often that won't be a problem. In fact, you will sometimes have the reverse task. Many patients are overly complimentary and initially have difficulty expressing concerns or dissatisfaction. To extract the maximum benefit for the learner, you may need to reiterate your invitation to the patient to express any difficulties that she experienced during the encounter. Your request will be reinforced if the learner echoes openness to being critiqued. You can also help the process by commending the patient when she makes constructive contributions. Still, for the rare patient who is unreasonably harsh or critical, you need to be prepared to interrupt the exchange and explain the limits of constructive feedback, or even terminate the session.

Consider withholding some of your feedback until you are alone with the learner. The review session with the patient is not a substitute for your review session with the learner. Your observations about the learner's performance, especially your negative comments, are best postponed until the two of you can meet privately. Even in the private session, you may want to invite the learner's further reflections before you offer your feedback. During the review session with the patient, your primary task is facilitating a meaningful dialogue between the patient and learner.

Before the review session with the patient ends, ensure that the patient is comfortable and arrange any needed follow-up. One possible side effect is that review sessions may have a negative impact on patients. Most patients with whom we've worked felt positively about their contributions to the learners' growth and indicated that they had learned from the session. But for some patients reviews can open previously unexplored worries and reawaken old sources of pain. So save time at the end of sessions for inviting patients to discuss their reactions, and ensure that they reach closure on any issues that have emerged. If a follow-up meeting or some additional form of care seems indicated, make sure that appropriate arrangements are made.

IN CONCLUSION

Patients are a potentially valuable source of feedback. The major task of health professionals is to be helpful to the people who turn to them for care, so it is essential to find out whether these people feel that they have indeed been helped. By routinely bringing patients into the learning process we can accomplish two important goals: We can help learners have access to this vital, unique source of information, and we can help learners develop a pattern that will have potential value throughout their careers.

Epilogue

If you were not convinced of the importance of fostering reflection and providing feedback before reading this book, we hope you are now. We hope you are also convinced that from the first days of their formal education, learners should be engaged in worthy experiences in classrooms, in patient care settings, and in the community. They should have opportunities—in real and simulated situations—to practice gathering information, thinking through clinical problems, eliciting information from patients, examining patients, searching the literature, applying new knowledge to the care of patients, presenting complex information to patients, doing procedures, collaborating with colleagues, and much more. Then they need opportunities to reflect on these experiences in the presence of teachers and peers and to invite the thoughts and feedback of these people. In addition, they need feedback from real and standardized patients.

In this book we presented numerous suggestions of steps to consider taking in fostering your learners' reflection and providing them with your reflections and feedback. We also suggested strategies for helping learners foster reflection and provide feedback to each other in small groups. Lastly we looked at ways to help learners elicit feedback from real and simulated patients. We hope these strategies will be of some practical use in your teaching.

We wrote this book for front-line educators. In doing so we didn't deal with an important, related issue: How can you do the kind of teaching we're recommending if you're working in a setting where people aren't likely to be open to these kinds of proposals? For example, we've acknowledged that it can be very difficult to foster reflection in a school or residency program that has a strongly competitive culture and devalues reflection. Influential people within institutions can directly challenge and even sabotage the work of educators who want to make changes. Protectors of the *status quo* are often in a position to simply deny would-be innovators the resources and political support they need.

Even if your institution devalues reflection and doesn't seek to give learners timely, constructive feedback from teachers, patients, and others, you can probably still foster reflection and provide helpful feedback in your own teaching. However, if you would like to help shift the climate of your school or program so reflection and feedback are more widely supported and practiced, what might you do other than get terribly frustrated?

Since innovators can get rapidly discouraged and be relatively ineffective if they feel isolated, a good first step is to find allies in your school or program, if you haven't already done so. We recommend that you meet whenever possible to reflect on your teaching and provide feedback and support to each other. You can also share ideas, goals, strategies, and reports from the educational literature.

As a group you might also want to consider how you can help bring about constructive changes in your system. For example, you might want to identify one or more influential leaders in your school who are reasonably open to the value of reflection and able to help you protect some time in the curriculum for reflection. Even a small step, such as bimonthly reflection groups for students who are working in the community, can have important symbolic and practical value.

You might also want to find support for including reflection and self-assessment among the behaviors on which students are evaluated in at least one or two courses. (The more courses the better, as students tend to resist changes in the evaluation system until they have a sufficient experience with the alternative to gain some familiarity and comfort, on their way to becoming defenders of the improved approach.)

Finding allies outside your institution can also be helpful. The Internet has become an excellent tool for helping educators find colleagues who share their interests and concerns. There are now a variety of ListServs through which educators raise questions and share ideas, strategies, and models. One of the first and most active is <dr-ed@list.msu.edu>, which is maintained by the Office of Medical Education Research and Development at Michigan State University. It provides a forum for lively exchanges among health professions educators. Some of the educators whose articles we've referenced in this book also can be sources of help and support. If you aren't already active in one of the many professional associations of educators in the health professions, we encourage you to explore these important sources of information, ideas, and opportunities for productive collaboration:

- Association of American Medical Colleges <www.AAMC.org>
- American Association of Colleges of Nursing
- Association of Physician Assistant Programs
- Association for Medical Education in Europe
- Society of Teachers of Family Medicine <www.stfm.org>
- The Network: Community Partnerships for Health through Innovative Education, Service, and Research <www.the-network.org>

The annual meetings of these and many other organizations provide exposure to a wide range of fresh insights and the possibility of learning from others who may have already tried some of the approaches you would like to consider.

We hope that you will be supported in any efforts you make to foster reflection and provide regular, constructive feedback in the teaching that you do. If you are already actively using these strategies, we imagine that you feel enriched as you watch your learners grow. If these approaches are new to you, we hope and anticipate that you will find fresh rewards for your efforts.

References

Angrist, S. W. (1973). *Closing the loop: The story of feedback.* New York: Thomas Y. Crowell.

Arendt, H. (1971). *The life of the mind. Vol. 1; Thinking.* San Diego, CA: Harcourt Brace Jovanovich.

Arseneau, R. (1995). Exit rounds: A reflection exercise. *Academic Medicine, 70,* 684–697.

Balint, M. (1972). *The doctor, his patient, and the illness.* New York: International University Press.

Barrows, H. S. (1985). *How to design a problem-based learning curriculum for the preclinical years.* New York: Springer.

Barrows, H. S., & Tamblyn, R. (1980). *Problem-based learning: An approach to medical education.* New York: Springer.

Black, N. M. I., & Harden, R. M. (1986). Providing feedback to students on clinical skills by using the Objective Structured Clinical Examination. *Medical Education, 20,* 48–52.

Botelho, F. J., McDaniel, S. H., & Jones, J. E. (1990). Using a family systems approach in a Balint-style group: An innovative course for continuing medical education. *Family Medicine, 22,* 293–295.

Boud, D., Keogh, R., & Walkers, D. (Eds.). (1985). *Reflection: Turning experiences into learning.* London: Kogan Page.

Boykin, A., & Schoenhofer, S. O. (1991). Story as link between nursing practice, ontology, and epistemology. *Image, 23*(4), 245–248.

Boykin, A., & Schoenhofer, S. O. (1993). *Nursing as caring: A model for transforming practice.* New York: NLN.

Brock, C. D., & Stock, R. D. (1990). A survey of Balint group activities in U.S. family practice residency programs. *Family Medicine, 22,* 33–37.

Butterfield, P. S., Mazzaferri, E. K., & Sachs, L. A. (1987). Nurses as evaluators of the humanistic behavior of internal medicine residents. *Journal of Medical Education, 62,* 842–849.

Charon, R., Banks, J. T., Connelly, J. E., Hawkins, A. K., Hunter, K. M., Jones, A. H., Montello, M., & Poirer, S. (1995). Literature and medicine: Contributions to clinical practice. *Annals of Internal Medicine, 122,* 599–606.

Collins, G. G., Cassie, J., & Daggett, C. (1978). The role of the attending physician in clinical training. *Journal of Medical Education, 53,* 429–431.

Cope, D. W., Linn, L. S., Leake, B. D., & Barrett, P. A. (1986). Modification of residents' behavior by preceptor feedback of patient satisfaction. *Journal of General Internal Medicine, 1*(6), 394–398.

DeTornyay, R., & Thompson, M. A. (1982). *Strategies for teaching nursing* (3rd ed.). New York: John Wiley & Sons.

Dewey, J. (1938). *Experience and education.* New York: Colliers Books.

Ende, J. (1983). Feedback in clinical medical education. *Journal of the American Medical Association, 250*(6), 777–781.

Epstein, R. M. (1999). Mindful practice. *Journal of the American Medical Association, 282*(9), 833–839.

Eron, L. D. (1955). Effect of medical education on medical students' attitudes. *Journal of Medical Education, 39*(10), 559–566.

Evans, C. E., Haynes, R. B., Gilbert, J. R., Taylor, D. W., Sackett, D. L., & Johnston, M. (1984). Educational package on hypertension for primary care physicians: Older physicians benefits most. *Canadian Medical Association Journal, 130,* 719.

Fischer, P. M. (1999). Evidentiary medicine lacks humility. *Journal of Family Practice, 48,* 345–346.

Franks, I. M., & Maile, L. J. (1991). The use of video in sport skill acquisition. In P. W. Dowrick (Ed.), *Practical guide to using video in the behavioral sciences* (pp. 231–243). New York: John Wiley & Sons.

General Professional Education of the Physician. (1984). *Physicians for the twenty-first century: Report of the project panel on the general professional education of the physician and college preparation for medicine.* Washington, DC: Association of American Medical Colleges.

Gil, D. H., Heins, M., & Jones, P. B. (1984). Perceptions of medical school faculty members and students on clinical clerkship feedback. *Journal of Medical Education, 59,* 950–952.

Glenn, J. K., Reid, J. C., Mahaffy, J., & Shurtleff, H. (1984). Teaching behaviors in the attending-resident interaction. *Journal of Family Practice, 18*(2), 297–304.

Gordon, M. J. (1991). A review of the validity and accuracy of self-assessments in health professions training. *Academic Medicine, 66,* 762–769.

Gordon, M. J. (1992). Self-assessment programs and their implications for health professions training. *Academic Medicine, 67,* 672–679.

Gordon, M. J. (1997). Cutting the Gordian knot: A two-part approach to the evaluation and professional development of residents. *Academic Medicine, 72*(10), 876–880.

Gordon, M. J. (1999). Commentary: Self-assessment skills are essential. *Education for Health, 12*(2), 167–168.

Hearnshaw, H., Baker, R., Cooper, A., & Soper, J. (1996). The cost and benefits of asking patients for their opinions about general practice. *Family Practice, 13,* 52–58.

Helfer, R. E. (1970). An objective comparison of the pediatric interviewing skills of freshman and senior medical students. *Pediatrics, 45*(4), 623–627.

Helfer, R. E., & Kempe, C. H. (Eds.). (1976). *Child abuse and neglect: The family and the community.* Cambridge, MA: Ballinger.

Henbest, R. J., & Fehrsen, G. S. (1985). Preliminary study at the Medical University of South Africa on student self-assessment as a means of evaluation. *Journal of Medical Education, 60,* 66–67.

Hewson, M., & Little, M. L. (1998). Giving feedback in medical education: Verification of recommended techniques. *Journal of General Internal Medicine, 13,* 111–116.

Irby, D. M. (1986). Clinical teaching and the clinical teacher. *Journal of Medical Education, 61*(9), 35–45.

Irby, D. M. (1995). Teaching and learning in ambulatory care settings: A thematic review of the literature. *Academic Medicine, 70,* 898–931.

Isaacson, J. H., Posk, L. K., Litaker, D. G., & Halperin, A. K. (1995). Resident perceptions of the evaluation process. Society of General Internal Medicine. *Journal of General Internal Medicine, 10*(Suppl.), 89.

Iverson, D. C., & Vernon, D. S. (1990). Program principles associated with successful health education and health promotion interventions. *Cancer Prevention, 1*(1), 43–50.

Jason, H., Kagan, N., Werner, A., Elstein, A., & Thomas, J. B. (1971). New approaches to teaching basic interviewing skills to medical students. *American Journal of Psychiatry, 127,* 1404–1407.

Jason, H., & Westberg, J. (1982). *Teachers and teaching in U.S. medical schools.* Norwalk, CT: Appleton Century-Crofts.

Johns, C., & Freshwater, D. (Eds.). (1998). *Transforming nursing through reflective practice.* Oxford, UK: Blackwell Science.

Kagan, N., & Kagan, H. (1991). Interpersonal process recall. In P. W. Dowrick (Ed.), *Practical guide to using video in the behavioral sciences* (pp. 221–230). New York: John Wiley & Sons.

Kahn, G., Cohen, B., & Jason, H. (1979). The teaching of interpersonal skills in U.S. medical schools. *Journal of Medical Education, 54,* 29–35.

Kaufman, A. (Ed.). (1985). *Implementing problem-based medical education: Lessons from successful innovations.* New York: Springer.

Kobert, L. J. (1995). In our own voice: Journaling as a teaching/learning technique for nurses. *Journal of Nursing Education, 34*(3), 140–142.

Kolb, D. A. (1984). *Experiential learning: Experience as the source of learning and development.* Englewood Cliffs, NJ: Prentice-Hall.

Kohn, L. T., Corrigan, J. M., & Donaldson, M. S. (Eds.). (2000). *To err is human: Building a safer health system.* Washington, DC: National Academy Press.

Lichstein, P. R. (1996). My most meaningful patient: Reflective learning on a a general medicine rotation. *Journal of General Internal Medicine, 11,* 406–409.

Linn, L. S., Oye, R. K., Cope, D. W., & DiMatteo, M. R. (1986). Use of non-physician staff to evaluate humanistic behavior of internal medicine residents and faculty members. *Journal of Medical Education, 61,* 918–920.

Lye, P., Bragg, D., & Simpson, D. (1997). Improving feedback with a clinical encounter form. *Academic Medicine, 72*(5), 444–445.

Lyons, J. (1999). Reflective education for professional practice; Discovering knowledge from experience. *Nurse Education Today, 9*(1), 29–34.

McCallum, J. (1987, April). Videotape is on a roll. *Sports Illustrated,* pp. 136–144.

McCue, J. D., Magrinat, G., Hansen, C. J., & Bailey, R. S. (1986). Residents' leadership styles and effectiveness as perceived by nurses. *Journal of Medical Education, 61,* 53–58.

McGrew, M., & Kaufman, A. (1999). Building blocks of innovation at the University of New Mexico. *Education for Health, 12*(1), 29–38.

McKegney, C. P. (1989). Medical education: A neglectful and abusive family system. *Family Medicine, 21*(6), 452–457.

Mezirow, J. (1998). On critical reflection. *Adult Education Quarterly, 48*(3), 185–198.

Nin, A. (1969). *The diary of Anais Nin, 1939–1944.* New York: Harcourt Brace & World.

Norcini, J. J., Shea, J. A., & Webster, G. D. (1986). Perceptions of the certification standards of the American Board of Internal Medicine. *Journal of General Internal Medicine, 1,* 166–169.

Novack, D. H., Suchman, A. L., Clark, W., Epstein, R. M., Najberg, E., & Kaplan, C. (1997). Calibrating the physician: Personal awareness and effective patient care. *Journal of the American Medical Association, 278*(6), 502–509.

O'Connor, F. W., Albert, M. L., & Thomas, M. D. (1999). Incorporating standardized patients into a psychosocial nurse practitioner program. *Archives of Psychiatric Nursing, 13*(5), 240–247.

O'Sullivan, P. S., Pinsker, J., & Landou, C. (1991). Evaluation strategies selected by residents: The roles of self-assessment, training level, and sex. *Teaching and Learning in Medicine, 3*(2), 101–107.

Papell, C. P., & Skolnik, L. (1992). The reflective practitioner: A contemporary paradigm's relevance for social work education. *Journal of Social Work Education, 28,* 18–26.

Pololi, L., Frankel, R. M., Clay, M., & Jobe, A. C. (2001). One year's experience with a program to facilitate personal and professional development in medical students using reflection groups. *Education for Health, 14,* 36–49.

Porter, L. (1982). Giving and receiving feedback; it will never be easy, but it can be better. *In National Training Lab Reading Book for Human Relations Training* (pp. 42–45). Bethel, ME: NTL.

Remmen, R., Denekens, J., Scherpbier, A., Hermann, I., van der Vleuten, C., Royen, P. V., & Bossaert, L. (2000). An evaluation study of the didactic quality of clerkships. *Medical Education, 34*(6), 460–464.

Riley-Doucet, D., & Wilson, S. (1997). A three-step method of self-reflection using reflective journal writing. *Journal of Advanced Nursing, 25*(5), 964–968.

Sackett, D. L., Haynes, R. B., & Gibson, E. S., Taylor, D. W., Roberts, R. S., & Johnson, A. L. (1977). Hypertension control, compliance and science. *American Heart Journal, 94*, 666–667.

Sackett, D. L., Haynes, R. B., & Tugwell, P. (1985). *Clinical epidemiology: A basic science for clinical medicine.* Boston: Little, Brown.

Scheidt, P. C., Lazoritz, S., Ebbeling, W. L., Figelman, A. R., Moessner, H. F., & Singer, J. E. (1986). Evaluation of a system providing feedback to students on videotaped patient encounters. *Journal of Medical Education, 61*, 585–590.

Schmidt, H. G., Magzoub, M., Feletti, G., Nooman, Z., & Vluggen, P. (Eds.). (2000). *Handbook of community-based education: Theory and practices.* Maastricht, the Netherlands: Network Publication.

Schön, D. A. (1983). *The reflective practitioner: How professionals think in action.* New York: Basic Books.

Schön, D. A. (1987). *Educating the reflective practitioner: Toward a new design for teaching and learning in the professions.* San Francisco, CA: Jossey-Bass.

Shapiro, J., & Lie, D. (2000). Using literature to help physician-learners understand and manage "difficult" patients. *Academic Medicine, 75*, 765–768.

Shatney, C. H., & Friend, B. E. (1984). Potential role of nurses in assessing house officer performance in the critical care environment. *Critical Care Medicine, 12*, 117–120.

Stillman, P. L., Regan, M. B., Philbin, M., & Haley, H. L. (1990). Results of a survey on the use of standardized patients to teach and evaluate clinical skills. *Academic Medicine, 65*, 288–292.

Stritter, F. T., Haines, J. D., & Grimes, D. A. (1975). Clinical teaching reexamined. *Journal of Medical Education, 50*, 876–882.

Stuart, M. R., Goldstein, H. S., & Snope, F. C. (1980). Self-evaluation by residents in family medicine. *Journal of Family Practice, 10*, 639–642.

Tannen, D. (1990). *You just don't understand: Women and men in conversation.* New York: William Morrow.

Thorndike, E. L. (1912). *Education.* New York: MacMillan.

Westberg, J., Kahn, G. S., Cohen, B., & Friel, T. (1980). Teaching interpersonal skills in physician assistant programs. *Medical Teacher, 1*, 136–141.

Westberg, J., & Jason, H. (1991). *Providing constructive feedback.* Boulder, CO: Center for Instructional Support.

Westberg, J., & Jason H. (1993). *Collaborative clinical education: The foundation of effective health care.* New York: Springer.

Westberg, J., & Jason, H. (1994a). Fostering learners' reflection and self-assessment. *Family Medicine, 26,* 278–282.

Westberg, J., & Jason, H. (1994b). *Teaching creatively with video: Fostering reflection, communication and other clinical skills.* New York: Springer.

Westberg, J., & Jason, H. (1996). *Fostering learning in small groups: A practical guide.* New York: Springer.

Whitman, N. (1993). A review of constructivism: Understanding and using a relatively new theory. *Family Medicine, 25,* 517–521.

Wigton, R. S., Kashinath, D. P., & Hoellerich, V. L. (1986). The effect of feedback in learning clinical diagnosis. *Journal of Medical Education, 61,* 816–822.

Wolverton, S., & Bosworth, M. (1985). A survey of resident perceptions of effective teaching behaviors. *Family Medicine, 17*(3), 106–108.

Wondrak, R., & Goble, J. (1992). An investigation into self, peer and tutor assessments of student psychiatric nurse's written work assignments. *Nurse Educator Today, 12*(1), 61–64.

Index